24 Hours to Save the NHS

24 Hours to Save the NHS

The Chief Executive's Account of Reform 2000 to 2006

Nigel Crisp

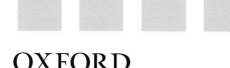

OXFORD
UNIVERSITY PRESS

OXFORD
UNIVERSITY PRESS

Great Clarendon Street, Oxford OX2 6DP

Oxford University Press is a department of the University of Oxford.
It furthers the University's objective of excellence in research, scholarship,
and education by publishing worldwide in

Oxford New York

Auckland Cape Town Dar es Salaam Hong Kong Karachi
Kuala Lumpur Madrid Melbourne Mexico City Nairobi
New Delhi Shanghai Taipei Toronto

With offices in

Argentina Austria Brazil Chile Czech Republic France Greece
Guatemala Hungary Italy Japan Poland Portugal Singapore
South Korea Switzerland Thailand Turkey Ukraine Vietnam

Oxford is a registered trade mark of Oxford University Press
in the UK and in certain other countries

Published in the United States
by Oxford University Press Inc., New York

British Library Cataloguing in Publication Data

Data available

Library of Congress Cataloging in Publication Data

Data available

Typeset by Newgen Imaging Systems (P) Ltd, Chennai, India
Printed in Great Britain
on acid-free paper by
Ashford Colour Press Ltd., Gosport, Hampshire

ISBN 978–0–19–963995–3

10 9 8 7 6 5 4 3 2 1

Whilst every effort has been made to ensure that the contents of this book are as complete, accurate and-
up-to-date as possible at the date of writing. Oxford University Press is not able to give any guarantee or
assurance that such is the case. Readers are urged to take appropriately qualified medical advice in all
cases. The information in this book is intended to be useful to the general reader, but should not be used
as a means of self-diagnosis or for the prescription of medication.

For Siân

Contents

Preface

What can we learn from your experience in England? I have been asked many times by ministers and health leaders around the world.

This book is an attempt to answer the question.

It is based on the implementation of the NHS Plan from 2000 which introduced a very comprehensive and far-reaching set of reforms into the NHS in England. It doesn't attempt to deal with every aspect of the reforms but, rather, to describe the perspective of the Chief Executive charged with running the service and making improvements. It is about making things happen as much as about policy.

After more than five and a half years running the NHS in England I have spent a similar period working in a number of countries around the world, mainly in Africa. Five years on from the NHS and with this added perspective, I have written an account that sets out the big picture and draws out some central themes.

I expect many readers will dip into the book: Chapters 1 and 3 provide the overview; Chapter 11 summarises the conclusions from the earlier chapters; and Chapters 12, 13 and 14 describe what I think are the implications today for England, other countries and global institutions respectively.

I hope that this account will provide some useful insights and contribute to the development of thinking about how best to promote health and deliver health services for people throughout the world.

Nigel Crisp
July 2011

Chapter 1

24 hours to save the NHS

24 hours to save the NHS. It was a political slogan, a final rallying cry for the Labour Party as it went into the General Election in May 1997. Their young new leader, Tony Blair, and his team were setting out the choice on offer in stark terms. There was a Labour commitment to keeping and strengthening the National Health Service whilst their Conservative opponents, Labour implied, would only dismember it, selling off its most profitable parts to their friends in the private sector.

They painted a picture of Labour preserving an NHS that was free for all as opposed to a Conservative free-for-all where the rich and powerful would, as always, come out on top. There was 24 hours to decide to vote Labour, they urged the country, and by doing so you could save the NHS.

Could the NHS survive?

Leaving the politics aside, there was a real question at the time about whether the British National Health Service could survive. Would this organisation, which offers free health care for every citizen regardless of their ability to pay, be able to survive and prosper in the 21st century? Was the extraordinary, liberating dream and ambition of its founders 50 years before – that everyone, no matter how poor or ill, should be freed from worrying about how to pay for their health care – still achievable?

This was a crucial issue at the end of the 20th century. The NHS had been in decline for some years with falling standards and failing public support and was the subject of endless media headlines deploring long waiting lists, denouncing shortages of staff and generally criticising its performance. Its friends were beginning to question its viability, whilst its enemies were eager to catalogue its faults.

Five years later we had an answer. Radical change and investment meant that the NHS had survived. Standards were improving and the NHS was expanding. Proof came from outside. Public satisfaction was increasing and had almost doubled by 2009.[1] Patients were voting with their feet with more people using the NHS and fewer people opting for private healthcare. This reversed the trend of recent years and forced the private sector in its turn to re-think its strategy.

Most tellingly, all the major political parties went into the 2010 general election committed to the NHS and to helping it develop and prosper. Public and political opinion had both changed.

Lessons for the future in the UK and elsewhere

The NHS was saved for the time being through a remarkable act of political will, followed through with major reforms and substantial extra funding. There are lessons and implications here for other countries both from what went well and from what didn't.

This account tells the story of reform and improvement in the biggest integrated health system in the world – the English NHS – with an annual budget today of more than £100 billion and 1.4 million directly employed staff, and which provides comprehensive services for 52 million people. It is the fourth biggest organisation of any sort in the world.[*]

It is a story of targeting improvement in priority areas: cutting waiting times for services dramatically, making it easier for people to get healthcare, reducing premature deaths from cancer and coronary heart disease, increasing staffing numbers and improving facilities.

It is not a straightforward tale. Reform was difficult even though there was a clear *NHS Plan*,[2] strong political leadership and substantial amounts of extra funding – all of which helped greatly but did not guarantee success.

It got off to an excellent start. Alan Milburn, the Secretary of State for Health who wrote the NHS Plan managed very skilfully to get the whole Government on board, secure the funding, buy in a wide range of stakeholders and launch the Plan in the best possible circumstances. This successful beginning created a momentum which was very helpful when policies were introduced later which took both the NHS and the Labour Party out of their comfort zones.

As Chief Executive I was responsible for implementing the Plan. We had failures along the way as well as achievements, faced opposition as we struggled to improve and had to learn how to implement our plans as we went along. There were no blueprints or maps to follow. Whilst we could – and did – learn elements from others there was an enormous amount that we had to create for ourselves.

There were a large number of people involved both in policy making and implementation and we didn't, of course, always agree amongst ourselves. There were some real differences of view and tensions both within the Department and across government. Despite this, we were able for 4 years or more to create a coherent leadership group of managers, politicians and clinicians and develop our own consistent approach. As a result we drove major reforms through the system and saw very significant improvements in patient care and health outcomes. Waiting times plummeted across the board, services improved and expanded, the NHS estate was rejuvenated and cancer and coronary heart disease survival rates improved massively.

---

[*] The Scots, Welsh and Northern Irish manage the NHS in their own countries and used the extra funding in different ways.

There were four areas of reform. In the first we concentrated on improving services by redesigning them. This meant, for example, speeding up treatment in the Accident and Emergency Department or making sure that when a patient needed some investigations they were able to get all their tests – bloods, X rays and so on – on the same visit to the hospital and didn't need to keep coming back for different things. We made sure that we learned these improvement techniques from the best organisations around the world.

Redesign of services, however, could only take us so far. We also needed to reform the way the system itself operated by changing organisational structures and incentives. We found that by decentralising, giving patients more choice and introducing some external competition we were able to accelerate improvement.

New services required new roles and new ways of working so the third area of reform was changing the way people worked in the NHS: restructuring the workforce and introducing new roles and new terms, conditions and pay in an effort to increase flexibility, effectiveness and efficiency.

The final reform was to make it easier for health workers to be certain what is the best treatment and improve the way knowledge, technology and science were used in the NHS.

The reforms themselves were very important: they were the designs for improvement and they excited and energised the planners and policy makers. Implementation, however, was a much grimmer affair and involved a relentless working through of the details; planning and adjusting plans as circumstances dictated.

Throughout the country there were clinicians and managers working very hard to deliver improvements one service at a time and one patient at a time. Nationally, my colleagues Neil McKay, John Bacon and Duncan Selbie could tell me at year end which patients had not been treated in time, which hospitals were not meeting targets and what was being done about it. John Reid, who took over as Secretary of State from Alan Milburn in 2003, recently told me that one of the things that stood out for him from this period was the sheer grind and the attention to detail that was needed to make large scale improvements.

There were literally thousands of people involved in the improvement efforts: it was their hard work that brought results. It was an extraordinarily tough time for people working in the NHS and I know that many disliked the targets and the pressure we put on the system. They also resented the times when policies seemed – and sometimes were – contradictory and the pace too fast.

I also remember, however, the celebrations which I witnessed in some hospitals when goals were achieved through people's own efforts – particularly when they had earlier seemed impossible and out of reach. We set a target reduction of 50% in the MRSA rate in the NHS in 2004 at a time when the best authorities said that we could only possibly achieve a 15% reduction. By 2011 it had fallen by 75%.[3]

Looked at objectively, there were very many successes and some failures.[4] I try to use external sources wherever possible in telling the story of the reforms. This book, however, is also an inside and subjective account of what it is like for a Chief Executive to be running a very large national health service whilst at the same time implementing a major reform programme which touched absolutely every part of the system. It deals with the pressures and contradictions of working with a wide range of stakeholders and politicians and offers an insight into how I tried – and sometimes failed – to steer the NHS on the most consistent and effective course.

Saved but not yet sustainable

The NHS may have been saved but it is not yet sustainable.

Like health systems in other western countries, the NHS faces enormous pressures as the population ages and costs grow. The NHS budget went up by 5.5% per year between 2000 and 2011 in real terms. It more than doubled over a ten year period from £49 billion to £103 billion between 2001 when the new money started to flow and 2011.[5]

The UK, however, still spends less than the European average on health as a percentage of GDP and even during the NHS Plan period its spending grew more slowly than spending in a number of similar countries.[6] We spend far less than the French (11.2% of GDP) and Germans (10.5%) both in overall terms and from public funds and, of course, far less than the Americans (16.0%). Nevertheless, at 8.7% of GDP in 2008 UK spend on healthcare is an enormous proportion of national expenditure.

It is perfectly reasonable to argue, of course, that healthcare spending will continue to rise as we get richer and that the population may well choose to spend more on health.[7] In any case, one might add, the UK can increase spending by 25% before it catches up with French and German expenditure. However, the real issue in today's straitened financial circumstances is what do we believe is sustainable and how should it be paid for.

There appear to be two schools of thought about what needs to be done to control growth in expenditure to a level that is both politically and fiscally possible and which will make the NHS sustainable in the long run.

The first, probably in the majority, see it as inevitable that in the words of a recent European study that consulted a number of health leaders: "*Keeping the universal healthcare model will require rationing of services and consolidation of healthcare facilities, as public resources fall short of demand.*"[8] This would have the implication that more healthcare would be paid for by individuals as opposed to from public funds and open up a wider market for private health care companies.

The second view is that growth in expenditure can be better managed through further reform. In order to serve our population better we need to transition from today's hospital and doctor based service models which deal primarily with treatment to new more community and people based ones concerned more with preventing disease and sustaining health. In doing so we need to extract some of the money tied up in our legacy of old infrastructure and working practices and transfer it to support the new services.

There is a great deal of agreement that, given the big increases in long term and chronic conditions in our aging population, we need to make this service change. In some form or other it has been part of Government policy in the UK and other countries for many years. The current Government, for example, wants GPs to drive just such a change.[9] There has been much less emphasis, however, on how this might help control spending growth.

Making such a change in the service model is enormously difficult, as the last 20 years and more have shown us. Health and research institutions, professional bodies, commercial organisations and thousands of individuals make their living from the old models. All would be at risk of losing power and income from such a change, most would resist it.

There is currently a pervading sense of inevitability about a move towards rationing and increased payments by patients which is epitomised by the study I referred to earlier. It is fostered in part, no doubt, by commercial and political interests who would gain from it by seeing a larger private market created. However, I also know that many health professionals who feel overwhelmed by their workload can see no other solution.

There is a choice here, however. We can chip away at the NHS, letting it drift back to the 90s with falling standards and failing services, or we can take on this enormous challenge and start to make decisive moves towards service changes and a sustainable future. The current Government is well placed to take up this challenge if it chooses to do so. There is a climate of austerity that favours decisiveness and it has the excellent platform of a much strengthened NHS to build on.

It is worth remembering what is at stake.

The founding values of the NHS as a service available equitably to everyone in the population are now contained in the NHS Constitution which has all party support.[10] This upholds the idea of the NHS as a social contract between citizen and state – where we expect our clinicians to do their best for us – and which is built on a solid basis of trust, relationships, attitudes, the passion of individuals and social capital.

There is a risk that as we tighten our belts financially we will erode this contract and reduce the NHS to providing a much smaller set of services and begin to see it as more of a commercial insurance contract with all the exclusions and limitations that that would entail.

Change at this scale will require political will and the ability to mobilise and motivate support. It will need to be well grounded intellectually in a good understanding of the current situation, future trends in health and the available evidence. I believe it will also need a re-definition of what the NHS is trying to accomplish in today's changed environment.

We need to move beyond our often sterile debates about public and private funding, demand management and the like and rephrase the fundamental problem as being about people and society and about how we want to live our lives.

We need to go beyond the managerial approach which achieved so much in the last 10 years, but we also need to go beyond the medical and professional model of looking at the world which has been the mainstay of the NHS since its inception. We need to keep the best aspects of both, of course; but most importantly we need to meet people where they are, integrate the NHS with other local services, break down barriers between the professions, and help people to have as much independence as possible to live "a life they have reason to live".

The closing chapters of this book set out how I think this can be done.

England and the world

I decided to write this book because so many ministers and senior health leaders in other countries asked me what they could learn from the English experience of reform. There are lessons here too for England today.

The NHS became a massive test bed for ideas during these reforms. Many different approaches, policies and designs were tried out at great scale and great speed and offer a rich source of ideas and experience – about what not to do as well as what to do – for politicians, policy makers and the public everywhere.

Many richer countries face similar problems to the UK and their solutions, subject to their culture and history, will doubtless need to be similar. My account of how we implemented reform in these four areas within a long established system will have some resonance and interest for them.

Most Commonwealth countries and several others modelled their own health systems on the NHS. This influence has been reinforced by the fact that so many doctors and nurses have either been educated and trained using British models in their own countries or actually in the UK. Here again I suspect there will be interest in how we have shaped and reshaped the NHS over the years whilst staying true to the founding values.

A large number of other countries including India and China – and covering more than half the world's population – are setting out to build and re-build health systems. South Africa and other African countries are recovering from past disasters and planning and making improvements. Brazil has an impressive track record in developing services for its population. There are parallels in all these countries with the way the NHS Plan set out to revive and revitalise the NHS and with the processes of implementation we adopted.

In many ways the most important point for those countries developing their health services is to avoid replicating the problems which countries like England with long established systems face. They need to ensure that they do not become dominated by the same institutions and interests as we are and end up creating a treatment and doctor dominated service. Many leaders in these countries understand this very well indeed and are trying to develop systems based on health and prevention of disease. They also recognise, however, how beguiling our models can be for the public and how powerful the global interests are that are promoting them.

Despite these pressures, new ideas about health and health systems are coming from all over the world. There is probably more creativity today in countries where they don't have our resources – or our baggage and vested interests – and are freer to try out new ideas and take risks, despite having far far worse problems than we do to contend with. Health is just like any other industry in this respect: many promising innovations come from emerging economies. There is a great deal we in the UK can learn.[11]

24 hours to save the NHS

This book has a very simple structure and readers can if they wish dip into it at any point.

Following this introduction, Chapter 2 sets out the national and global context dealing with the foundation of the NHS in 1948, its decline at the end of the 20th century and the global trends which will affect its future.

Chapter 3 gives a brief account of the reforms: telling the story of what happened primarily between 2000 and 2006 but with some updating to the present day.

The next four chapters, 4 to 7, each address one of the areas of reform: service redesign, system reform, workforce restructuring and knowledge, technology and science. These chapters describe what we tried to do in these areas and identify the lessons for the future.

The next three chapters each tackle a major cross cutting issue. Chapter 8 deals with finance and productivity and with what it might mean for the NHS to become financially sustainable. Chapter 9 is the most personal chapter and discusses leadership and in particular how I approached my role as Chief Executive of the NHS and Permanent Secretary of the Department of Health, and coped with the many and conflicting pressures which were involved. Chapter 10 deals with patients and society and the way we tried to help them to take up their proper role at the centre of health and healthcare.

The final four chapters are about the future. Chapter 11 draws together the conclusions and key points from earlier chapters. Chapter 12 addresses the future of the NHS in England and contains my assessment of the Coalition Government's proposed reforms and my view about how the NHS in England could become sustainable and thrive in the future. Chapter 13 describes what I believe are the lessons for the rest of the world from the NHS Plan and its reforms, Chapter 14 concludes with some short observations about the global action that is necessary to continue to improve health worldwide.

There are four appendices at the end of the book: a glossary of terms, a simple description of NHS structure, a time line of events and the "must do" targets from the NHS Plan.

The Chief Executive's account of reform

This book is written from the standpoint of the Chief Executive charged with simultaneously running the NHS in England and the Department of Health for the whole of the UK.

This account does not aspire to be objective or comprehensive, but is intended to be both accurate and truthful. It is my perspective and offers a unique and subjective view of the period. It uses data where this is available from reputable sources. I have also checked the references I have made to them with most of those mentioned, some of whom have also provided me with their own memories and reflections.

Whilst I am not a member of any political party I am unashamedly partisan about the NHS. I want it to work and have spent the most active 20 years of my life from my mid 30s to my mid 50s working for the NHS under different Governments and trying to improve it. I am not however – as will be obvious from the following chapters – blind to its faults. It needs further reform and improvement.

Throughout those 20 years I have set aside time to walk the wards, visit the departments and ask permission from patients and clinicians to go into operating theatres and surgeries. In my later regional and national roles I adopted the habit of doing this every Friday. I have visited very nearly every major hospital in the country and GPs' surgeries in every county. This gave me the chance to see, listen to and talk with patients and NHS staff and to ask questions. It provided me with the visual and aural evidence to go with the paperwork and figures I saw and could act as a counter weight to the sometimes over optimistic or over gloomy accounts I was given by others.

It was also rather therapeutic. After the early part of my week had been spent with Ministers and dealing with crises and all sorts of alarms and excursions it was reinvigorating to meet health workers and patients, to see what was happening, to comment and applaud and sometimes, sadly, to be shocked by what I saw or heard. It reminded me of what it was all about and it provided NHS staff with the opportunity to discuss issues and challenge me face to face and on their own territory.

Sometimes insights come from places that you might not expect.

Even if I hadn't seen things for myself I would have been kept honest by Judy Sweeting who was my driver throughout my time as Chief Executive. Judy is a very direct person who would go into the hospital or clinic anonymously after she had dropped me at the front door to be greeted by the Chair or Chief Executive. She carried out her own inspection. She would sit in the canteen or a waiting room, walk around the buildings and observe unnoticed.

Later, like all good interrogators, she would get the first question in as she drove me away. What did I think of the hospital?

"*Well it seemed quite good*", I would reply hesitatingly, guessing what was to come.

"That's not what the patients say" she would respond firmly. "You ought to have heard what they said about the wards".

Sometimes, of course, there were warm words of praise.

It kept me honest. I was reminded of the importance of having people around me who told me the truth.

Conclusions and key points

1. In 2000 there was real doubt as to whether the NHS could survive. It did so thanks to a major act of political will, radical reforms and massively increased funding. Public satisfaction almost doubled, patients returned from the private sector and a new political consensus about maintaining the NHS was established.

2. Action was centred on the NHS Plan which targeted improvements in priority areas including cutting waiting times for services dramatically, making it easier for people to get healthcare, reducing premature deaths from cancer and coronary heart disease, increasing staffing numbers and improving facilities.

3. There were four main areas of reform:
   a. Service redesign and improvement
   b. System reform
   c. Restructuring the workforce
   d. Knowledge, technology and science.

4. The design of the reforms was very important but implementation also required a relentless working through of the details; planning and adjusting plans as circumstances dictated.

5. The NHS may have been saved but it is not yet sustainable. There is once again a need for a radical approach which will enable the NHS to transition from a service focussed on hospitals, doctors and disease treatment to one which is community based, people centred and geared towards prevention and promotion.

Conclusions and key issues (*Continued*)

6. The NHS needs to develop a new approach that goes beyond managerialism and the medical model, keeping the best aspects of both, meeting people where they are and supporting them in how they want to live their lives.

7. There are many lessons here for the NHS in the future and for other countries both about the design of reforms and about implementation. The UK can also learn from other countries including those which don't have our resources, or our baggage and our vested interests, and are freer to innovate.

References

1. National Centre for Social Research (2010) *British Social Attitudes 27th Report.*
2. Department of Health (2000) *The NHS Plan – a plan for investment, a plan for reform*; Cmd 4818-1, The Stationary Office.
3. Health Protection Agency. *Results from the mandatory surveillance of MRSA bacteraemia;* monthly figures.
4. Healthcare Commission. *State of Healthcare in England and Wales 2008;* December 2008.
5. Department of Health: financial allocations.
6. OECD Health data 2010.
7. Baumol WJ (1993) Social wants and dismal science: the curious case of the climbing costs of health and teaching. *Proc Am Philos Soc* **137**: 612–37.
8. Economist Intelligence Unit: *The future of healthcare in Europe;* 2011.
9. UK Government: *Health and Social Care Bill, 2010–2011.*
10. Department of Health: *The NHS Constitution;* 300635 8 March 2010.
11. Crisp N (2011) *Turning the World Upside Down – the search for global health in the 21st century;* RSM Press.

Chapter 2

The national and global context

Even as the Chief Executive of the hospital there appeared to be very little I could do about it.

We had a major problem in the Accident and Emergency Department (A and E) in Oxford in the 1990s. So many people arrived in A and E each day that we had great trouble coping. On many evenings we had patients, sometimes very ill and almost always in distress, waiting on trolleys in corridors to be seen or to be admitted. It was awful for patients, their relatives and for staff.

The John Radcliffe (JR) sits at the centre of a number of smaller hospitals which between them cover a population of about a million in Oxfordshire and neighbouring counties. Each provides general services and some specialist care for their local population but each also relies on the JR and the other Oxford teaching hospitals to provide the most specialist services – heart surgery, kidney transplant, paediatric intensive care and the like – and, in the case of the JR, to take their emergency overflow when they got too busy.

The A and E Department at the JR – and its patients – suffered from being the crucial back up not only for its own hospital but also for the whole surrounding area. The difficulty was not so much seeing and assessing the patients but finding a bed for those who needed admission. Nurses had a constant battle to persuade their colleagues on the wards to take patients from A and E. Sometimes ward staff couldn't admit patients because they were genuinely full but sometimes they refused because they were reserving space for the next day's surgery intake and didn't want to cancel operations. Tensions could develop with accusations of territorialism and deceit. It was stressful and unhealthy.

There was very little I could do to affect the flows of patients to the hospital and I had no money to open more beds or create larger facilities. As a Management Team, however, we decided that we needed to become personally involved and so we established a rota to go into A and E each evening and use our own authority to ease the situation, move people and find extra resources wherever we could. It worked after a fashion: we dealt with blockages, talked to Consultants and, as importantly as anything, offered explanations to patients and support for staff.

The truth was, however, that we were just fire fighting. It was deeply frustrating to be so powerless. It was a feeling I know I shared with the Consultants and senior nurses in the hospital – and it motivated me very strongly when I later had the chance as Chief Executive of the NHS to help drive improvements in all our A and E Departments.

I could have started this chapter with some of the many good stories I heard as Chief Executive of the hospital about the wonderful care people were shown, about the near miracle improvements, or the skills of the staff or even how easy the hospital had made it for a relative in their last days. I heard all of these from patients and their families on a regular basis. Re-telling them here, however, would not be so instructive. It was the problems and the difficulties that drove improvement and led to the decisive action by Government to review the NHS and establish the NHS Plan.

The starting point for reform

This chapter provides the national and global context for the NHS Plan: the starting point for reform. It begins with patients and the reality of working in the NHS in the 1990s when performance was poor and resources tight before going on to look at national politics and the history of the NHS since its foundation in 1948. It considers the internal dynamics of the NHS and the role and power of clinicians and other staff and concludes with a discussion of the global health trends that are already affecting us.

The problems patients and staff experienced in Oxford were not unique and were very far from being the worst in the country. Too many A and E Departments felt like battle zones with the injured and sick waiting around for treatment. A number of patients' organisations responded by identifying the worst cases and publicising the occasions when people stayed 24 hours, 36 hours or even 48 in a Department. These so-called "trolley waits" became, rightly, a cause célèbre in the media.

The most visible problems at that time were almost always about hospitals: A and E Departments featured regularly but so did long waiting times, staff shortages and ward closures. There were also stories about delays in ambulances reaching patients and about people being discharged prematurely from mental health units.

Inner cities and London in particular had problems in primary care with run down GP premises, large numbers of unregistered patients – some migrants, some moving house, and some simply living chaotic lives – and high levels of deprivation. This led to many complaints about the time it took to see a GP in these areas and criticisms of always seeing different staff, many of them temporary. There was much more variation in the standard of primary care from practice to practice and place to place than there was between hospitals. Some practices were absolutely wonderful, some were unbelievably dire.

Part of the problem was about resources. The UK, which had spent a similar proportion of GDP on health to France and other European countries in 1960, had fallen behind over the succeeding years so that by 1999 France spent 10.1% of

GDP on health, Germany 10.3% and the UK only 6.9%.[1] This was reflected in staffing figures – with the UK having 1.9 doctors per 1,000 population and France and Germany each 3.3 in 2000[2] – and in outdated facilities and poor levels of equipment. In the NHS Plan it was estimated that a third of its buildings dated from before the foundation of the NHS 52 years earlier and that there was a £3.1 billion backlog maintenance problem.[3]

By 2000 even the Treasury was beginning to recognise that the NHS needed extra funding and in the Wanless Report of 2002 expressly granted additional funding to "catch up" for the years of lost investment and recognised that there would be falls in productivity whilst this happened.[4] The NHS was trying to do the same job as health systems in other countries in Europe with typically only about 70% of the money.

Systems and "the system"

However, systems, processes and working practices were another major part of the problem.

Hospitals were too full for several reasons: there were patients, cruelly called "bed blockers", who were ready for discharge but had nowhere they could safely go; there were unnecessary admissions because there were no alternatives available in the community; and there were often avoidable delays in discharging patients. A and E Departments themselves had their own system problems with delays in access to X rays and pathology tests, poor staff deployment systems and bottle necks over access to equipment. The primary care problems were frequently to do with the location of practices – with fewer in the poorest and most needy areas – inadequate premises and poor staff rostering.

Systems were to become a key theme of the NHS reforms with the recognition that improving systems was absolutely central to improving healthcare. It was not, as we had found in Oxford, about working harder but – in the cliché – about "working smarter" to improve systems. If we could do something about the patients whose discharges were delayed or speed up path lab results or X rays we would start to see real improvements.

These were not purely management and organisational issues but often reflected the way health workers had been trained and were regulated. Nurses couldn't generally order X rays for patients but had to wait for the doctor to do so, individual clinicians made their own sometimes quite personal decisions about when patients were ready for discharge without any agreed protocols and the different specialities had their own junior staff who were not able to treat patients who hadn't been referred to their speciality, even if they had already trained in the relevant area. I came across absurd situations where GPs had to refer patients to orthopaedic surgeons in order to get physiotherapy, rather than referring directly to the physiotherapist. Professional demarcation was rife.

There were also problems with incentives. In a system where hospitals have fixed budgets they have no financial incentives to treat more patients and reduce waiting times. Instead, perversely, there were incentives for Consultants to have a long waiting list in the NHS — where their salaries were fixed regardless of how much work they did — so that more patients would choose to become private patients and pay the Consultant to operate on them.

It is easy to see in these circumstances why front line staff, without any authority other than over the patient in front of them so often felt they were battling "the system", trying to find ways round it to give their patients what was needed or to exercise some control over their work flow. This powerlessness was one of the biggest sources of stress and poor morale.

It is even easier to see why patients felt baffled when things don't happen as they thought they should — why couldn't we guarantee there was going to be a bed for them to come into for their operation in the morning, why couldn't the nurse — who seemed to know much more than the junior doctor — prescribe the tablets or discharge them, why did the different professions keep different sets of notes, why couldn't the Consultant talk to the GP directly?

Later I would see Ministers and even a Prime Minister frustrated by the same web of issues and contradictions.

These sorts of problems are not limited to the NHS in England or even to the UK and I suspect health workers from other countries will recognise most of them — and could add additional ones of their own.

The need for radical reform not incremental change

The NHS has many very good systems, of course, built into its basic structure. It is funded by general tax and there is a single payer. Funding is allocated to NHS organisations which cover geographical populations on the basis of population size weighted for socio-economic factors and local market conditions. Each of us is expected to register with a General Practitioner (GP) who refers us on for elective care and consultation and we can get emergency treatment in any NHS facility in the country. Appendix 2 gives a fuller description of the NHS.

This is simply what we expect in the UK and we probably take these advantages for granted. This structure avoids many processes that others have to endure — we don't have to find (or, indeed, pay for) insurance cover, check which hospitals are available to us, make sure the clinician's proposed treatment is covered, arrange our own referrals and pay the bills. There are some weaknesses, of course, about choice and range of services which the NHS Plan reforms sought to address. However, there is no doubt that these NHS processes are simpler and cheaper than many others. This is reflected, for example, in the fact that NHS overheads and bureaucratic processes are less than half the cost proportionately of the US system.[5]

The truth was that by 2000, however, the NHS was performing poorly, gave an inadequate service to many of its patients and was in decline. It was not just in funding that we compared badly with our neighbours – cancer survival rates, the numbers of heart attacks and patient satisfaction scores all compared badly with the results from France, Germany and many comparator countries.

Moreover, as some of the examples given in this chapter show, there was a lack of unity and direction. Different parts of the system and different groups of staff were pulling in different directions. There was a sense of drift as well as of the helplessness I had felt in Oxford. This was a health system in – possibly terminal – decline.

The scale of the problems demanded radical and national action if the NHS were to survive. Many people were as frustrated as I had been in Oxford that they couldn't tackle problems that affected them but went outside their authority. They could only deal with some of the issues.

As a hospital Chief Executive I had only very limited influence on the numbers of emergency patients coming to the JR from the surrounding area. Later as a Regional Director and responsible for a large part of the country I could have some influence on patient movements across the whole area but I couldn't change the incentives which, as I described earlier, often interfered with providing the best patient care. Even as the Chief Executive of the whole NHS in England I could do very little about the funding issues other than argue the case for more money. Unlike other industries we couldn't earn more by providing more services. Ultimately I needed the paymaster, Parliament, to vote the money.

There needed to be a very large scale national solution which tackled the problems at every level from service design to reform of incentives and staffing structures.

This needed a major act of political will.

The founding of the NHS

Let me return to the beginning and briefly set today's issues in the context of NHS history.

The founding of the NHS was a profoundly political act in 1948, part of the creation of a Welfare State which aspired to look after its citizens *from cradle to grave*. It was part of the new future for a country re-building itself after the Second World War. Health care was to be comprehensive, available equally to everyone, rich and poor alike. Because it was paid for by taxes it would be *free at the point of need*.[6]

Similar developments in recent years in countries in Asia, Africa and South America are also profoundly political and part of building a new vision of their nation, whether in newly democratic Cambodia or Ethiopia, post apartheid South Africa or the rapidly expanding economies of Brazil, China and India.

I have heard Dr Aaron Motsoaledi, South African Minister of Health and a veteran of "the struggle", talk passionately about providing healthcare for people who have long been oppressed under apartheid. I have also heard people who are not politicians such as Francis Omaswa, formerly Director General of Health Services in Uganda and now active in many global health ventures, remind international audiences that it is "our" people who are suffering and dying from national and international neglect. There are echoes here of the sentiments and language of the politicians and other leaders – the Bevans and the Beveridges – who created the NHS.

All politics divides as well as unites. The creation of the NHS was supported by many including, of course, most of the people who would have access to regular healthcare for the first time. It was also opposed by many. The issue was largely a question of how people saw the world and what they believed to be the role of the state and of government. It complicated and was, in turn, complicated by politics and ideology. The doctors' organisation, the British Medical Association, opposed the founding of the NHS although, as we shall see later in this chapter, this was out of self-interest.

More recently we have seen very similar divisions in the United States as President Obama and his supporters have fought to introduce and implement reforms which, amongst other things, provide a minimum insurance cover for all its citizens. These reforms have become a focus for division across the nation. Here too it is about world view and perceptions of the role of government. Amongst the less extreme assertions are that it is un-American and un-constitutional to impose health insurance on free citizens, on the one hand, and that it is immoral and against the laws of natural justice not to provide cover for everyone on the other.

These reforms unlike the 1948 British ones have been supported by the doctors' organisation, the American Medical Association. It is rumoured to have lost a third of its membership as a direct result.

The NHS was established at the end of the Second World War as part of a much wider set of social changes which included two new Education Acts which created new schools and extended the school leaving age; and a new Social Security system which extended the range and the amount of benefits paid for unemployment, sickness and disability. These changes, in the words of Sir William Beveridge who wrote the definitive report on which they were based, were intended "*to slay the 5 giants of want, disease, ignorance, squalor and idleness which stalk the land*".[7,8]

The NHS was only one part of the creation of the Welfare State at the end of the war when the nation began re-building itself to a very different design from the pre-war model. Looking back it is possible to see how a whole range of reforming movements dating back over many years – and involving wider voting rights, with women getting the vote in 1921, the first pension entitlements for some groups of men in 1911 and the establishment of compulsory education in 1878 – culminated in this broad and deep package of reforms in the late 1940s. The progress was not linear but the direction was consistent.

Each of these reforms complimented the others with the health of the population, for example, improved by better education, pension and unemployment provision. This was about building a better country for its citizens. This is the same as the position today in large parts of Africa or Asia, Latin America, India or China where governments work to deliver integrated plans to defeat poverty and improve health and education. The five giants walked together in the UK in 1948, as they do in many parts of the world in 2011; but so, too, do the giant slayers.

Two points from its foundation stand out that are immediately relevant to our story. The first is that the NHS was born with a compromise at its heart which still has implications today. The original plan was to nationalise the hospitals and employ the doctors and all other health workers within a national service. Aneurin Bevan, the Secretary of State for Health faced resistance. He was able to overcome any opposition from the hospital authorities but was resisted strongly by the doctors who, as always, had powerful allies.

It is very interesting to read Bevan's speeches of the time in which he sets out his vision for the NHS to a variety of different medical and other audiences around the country. As time progresses his position begins to change as he modifies his negotiating position. There were many twists and turns, plots and sub-plots, in the story of the founding of the NHS.[9]

The result, the final compromise, was that the hospitals were nationalised but the doctors won two important victories. The first was that the hospital specialists, the Consultants, became employees of the NHS Regions rather than of the individual hospitals and, crucially, retained their right to do private practice in their non-NHS time. The second was that the GPs remained independent practitioners who had service contracts rather than employment contracts with the NHS.

The consequences of this compromise are profound. It allowed the doctors to have a very great say in the organisation without a great deal of accountability. It meant that the NHS was presented with a firm barrier between hospital and community care based not on any kind of principle about how services might best be organised but simply on a negotiation with a trade union. It also meant that the boundaries between public and private healthcare were blurred. Many would-be reforming ministers have over the years tried to tackle each of these issues, legacies of this early compromise. Bevan himself was unhappy about it and is said to have talked of having to *stuff the doctors' mouths with gold* to get them to cooperate with the NHS. Other ministers have subsequently found themselves doing the same thing.

The second major point is that the NHS was born of a particular time and culture and, like the whole Welfare State, has found it very difficult to adapt as times and the external environment have changed.

There was controversy and opposition to its foundation but for a long period there was a broad consensus of support. It was a source of comfort and passion for the very many people who would be able for the first time to be free from worrying about how to pay for healthcare and escape the dreadful fear that illness might lead their whole family to penury and the workhouse. For members of the Labour movement it was iconic. John Reid, one of the Secretaries of State I worked with, described it as *"the greatest gift the British people have ever given themselves"*. For many others it was a sign of British civilisation and a gift we handed on to the world through the Commonwealth. There was even a sense that it was *"the envy of the world"*.

The NHS was established at much the same time as other welfare states and social benefit structures across Europe. These are all built on a sense of social solidarity and of some shared values which run very deep. They represent social contracts between the citizen and the state and are about citizens' rights and expectations. They are very different from health insurance schemes which are based on commercial contracts and offer only consumers' rights and protections.

TR Reid, the Washington Post journalist, writes of visiting the Swiss Minister of Finance and asking him innocently how many people went bankrupt each year in Switzerland as a result of the cost of healthcare. Reid knew that 4% of bankruptcies each year were due to healthcare costs in his own country. Reid has made a film of his book which includes this interview. In it we see the Minister pausing for a moment as though in surprise and then replying *"No one of course. It would be immoral."*[10]

This illustrates both the trans-Atlantic gulf on this issue and the depth of European assumptions about healthcare available to all. It is the answer of someone who sees healthcare as being part of a social contract and not just something bought through an insurance scheme or paid for by individuals.

Failure to thrive and adapt

Despite its success the NHS failed to adapt as society changed and the political climate in the 70s and 80s moved against it. I remember being told by Anne Ferguson, a marketing director at ICI Paints in the early 90s and a non-executive director of my hospital, how successful ICI had been in introducing very small amounts of different colours into white paint so as to produce subtly different shades. They had multiplied sales of that basic commodity, white paint, many times as a result. "*Nigel*", she said, "*if the public wants personalised white paint they will certainly want personalised health care*".

Yet we weren't giving it to them. The NHS as a system was still too often treating patients in groups, not giving appointment times, not offering some of the basic "customer care" we were getting from our banks or other businesses and failing, all too frequently, to make us feel valued as human beings. Individual staff members and clinicians may have been wonderful but the overall effect was not.

I also remember my Chairman at Wexham Park and Heatherwood Hospitals, Sir Brian Smith, asking at the same period why the main entrance of the hospital looked like the entrance to a scruffy benefit office. "*Weren't we proud of what we were doing?*" I didn't think to ask why a benefit office needed to be scruffy. I suppose it must have been what I expected of the buildings of the Welfare State by that stage in its development.

It was obvious that the NHS – like the rest of the Welfare State – was in trouble. The Conservatives, who were in government throughout the 80s and most of the 90s, had, at best, an ambivalent attitude towards the NHS. Their Secretaries of State were clearly personally working for improvement but the organisation was starved of funds and the subject of much political sniping and criticism. Public concern about the NHS led Mrs Thatcher as Prime Minister to hold an NHS review and introduce changes. Three significant reforms were brought in during the years when she and, subsequently, Sir John Major were Prime Ministers.

General Managers were appointed in 1985 to take personal responsibility for the operation of units following a report from Sir Roy Griffiths who in a famous description said "*if Florence Nightingale were carrying her lamp through the corridors of the NHS today she would almost certainly be searching for the people in charge.*"[11] I joined the NHS in 1986 as a "*Griffiths manager*" appointed from a career elsewhere to run a Mental Handicap hospital and unit – nowadays it would be described as a Learning Difficulties Service.

This was the start of the rise of managerialism in the NHS, with further developments over the next few years leading to a much more managed and accountable system. This was followed by a policy for "*the separation of purchasers and providers*" which for the first time created a division in the NHS between those organisations – at that time Health Authorities – which had responsibility for the health of a whole population, and the hospitals and other units which were mainly providers of services. Health Authorities became the funder or purchaser of services from hospitals and other providers. This split was designed both to ensure that funding decisions were not made in the interests of the providers and that the provider units would have a financial incentive to meet the purchaser's requirements.

This radical change was accompanied by the creation of NHS Trust Hospitals in 1991 as semi-autonomous units within the NHS which were designed to ensure better local management and accountability and enable them to become better providers of services. For the first time, following the 1948 compromise, Consultants became employees of the hospital where they worked.

The creation of NHS Trusts was seen as a very political act and, from the left, as a prelude to selling off or privatising the hospitals. It became a focus of the 1992 General Election. As the General Manager of an acute hospital at the time which was aspiring to become an NHS Trust I well recall the political rancour caused in a tight fought election which the Conservatives won against the run of the polls. We were able to go ahead with our plans.

These changes were not as effective as they might have been because the separation of purchaser and provider and the semi-autonomous status of the Trust Hospitals were not established in law. This meant that Ministers and the NHS centrally were always able to overrule local agreements and step in with their own decisions. This was widely resented by Boards and Chief Executives across the country who had thought that they had much more freedom of action.

The critics were right to the extent that these three reforms paved the way for the later market reforms under Labour, which gave purchasers and Trusts the authority they wanted in law. Whilst not privatisation, this was a very substantial change in the way the NHS worked which began a process of moving it from being, in effect, a nationalised industry – with centralised structures and authority – to becoming a national health system, with more diversity and greater local autonomy.

There is a remarkable continuity of policy here, despite all the politics and the organisational changes over the years. It can be seen very clearly in retrospect. The Conservative Government of 1979–1997 laid the foundations which were built on by Labour from 1997 to 2010 and which are now being developed further by the Coalition Government once more. The other remarkable continuity of policy throughout this period is the emphasis on primary care and, as it was called in 1994 a *"Primary Care Led NHS"*. This policy is an important part of our story and the role of primary care as gatekeeper, purchaser and commissioner will figure large in the remainder of the book.

If the Conservatives were ambivalent at the time, Labour seemed simply to be against change, any change. Any tinkering with the NHS appeared to be seen as tantamount to the destruction of the NHS. More money was the answer whatever the question. Even on entering government in 1997, and despite the election rhetoric, Labour started to tackle the problems in health rather slowly. There was a sense that it didn't feel there was very much that it needed to do to change the system and that by steering it wisely, providing more money and working with the staff the necessary improvements would come.

This slow start was evident in other parts of government, perhaps not surprising after so many years in opposition.

The really radical changes started in 2000 with the launch of the NHS Plan and in 2001 when the money to fund it began to be available. The Labour Party had moved on enormously in these few years. I recall John Reid, Secretary of State from 2003 to 2005, saying, in an interesting echo of Anne Ferguson's remarks of 10 years before, "*In 1948 it was like Henry Ford saying you could have any colour of car you wanted as long as it was black, people were simply delighted to have a health service. Now, just as you now really can have any colour of car you want, people want personalised care and attention*".

The NHS is still working through the legacy of its 1948 founding. It and the Welfare State are both changing and the new Government is clearly determined to leave its impact on both. It is interesting to see how both main political parties are struggling with their own ideas of the Big Society and the Good Society as some sort of re-framing or replacement of the Welfare State. The evolution of the NHS has some way still to go.

Similarly, the results of the compromise with the doctors are still being played out through the system.

Culture, clinicians and power

Culture in the very broad sense of how people think and behave is a very important issue and will be returned to time and again throughout this account.

NHS culture at first sight seems wonderful. We all know of caring staff working in a system that cares about each one of us and I, like other patients, am very grateful for the way I have been looked after in the NHS. There are thousands of people working in the NHS who embody its values, focus on the needs of each patient and strive to keep themselves up to date with the latest knowledge. There is still a clear sense that the doctor will do his or her best to help you and that the nurse will always be on your side.

Moreover many students and young professionals, as I know from my regular contact with them, are strongly driven by a desire to do something worthwhile in the world and to "make a difference" with their lives.

The downside to these strong motivations is, as we shall see shortly, that clinicians can become too powerful and controlling and leave little room for other ideas to develop and for patients' own views and decisions to be heard. Closer inspection also reveals that as well as these very positive cultural features there are many sub-cultures and some deep rooted attitudes and behaviours which can cause enormous problems for patients and the population as well as for staff.

Rosabeth Moss-Kanter of Harvard has pointed out that not all health workers want the same thing. There are tensions between different groups and one group's gain may be another's loss:

> "*Supposedly, everyone working in health care wants the same thing: to help people get and stay healthy. 'Everyone' includes primary care doctors, medical specialists, nurses, hospital administrators, health insurance providers, nutritionists, pharmaceutical companies, medical technology manufacturers, fitness gurus, paraprofessionals, public health commissioners, and charities dedicated to a disease.*
> *The problem is that everyone can have a different view of the meaning of getting and staying healthy. Lack of consensus among players in a complex system is one of the biggest barriers to innovation. One subgroup's innovation is another subgroup's loss of control.*"[12]

These differences of perspectives can have profound implications and are very important in understanding the history of the NHS and how it has developed over the years. There are many subplots to uncover: how doctors and nurses have struggled over professional boundaries; how midwives and obstetricians have done the same; how, even, the different branches of medicine such as radiology and surgery have disagreed about who should undertake which procedures and, most recently, how the introduction of professional managers disrupted the existing balance of powers.

As Rosabeth Moss-Kanter describes, these struggles have always been, ostensibly at least, over the different groups' interpretations of what is best for the patient. They have also, as her quotation makes clear, made it harder to introduce innovation because one group's gain is another's loss.

Increasingly in recent years politicians have also entered the fray with their own interpretation of what may be best for the patient or population. There is often a fine line here between what is seen as clinically desirable and what is politically appropriate. Just such a case occurred with the introduction of the Mental Health Act, finally passed in 2007, which attempted to balance the rights of people with mental illness and the State's duty to protect the citizen. Many mental health professionals believed that it went too far in restricting the rights of the individual in the interest of the wider public and therefore campaigned hard against it. The politicians maintained their view of what they saw as the right balance for society.

Sometimes science, research and evidence can resolve these issues satisfactorily but in many cases there is room for different sorts of interpretations and, therefore, potential disagreement and struggle.

Culturally, there have been three broad shifts in relationships and power over the years since the foundation of the NHS. The first involves the medical profession and other groups. Doctors, who at the start of the NHS were all-powerful, have seen others take on wider and more powerful clinical as well as organisational roles. Politicians, too, have become more involved in the detail of policy.

Many examples can be pointed to, from nurses being allowed to prescribe drugs to the introduction of general managers and chief executives in charge of institutions and services. All of them appear to take away something from the doctor's role. Moreover, as Atul Gawande and others have argued, the sheer complexity of modern healthcare means that doctors have to be more reliant on their teams and other people.

A famous story from 2000 illustrates how some doctors have felt about this. It recounts that a group of senior doctors had just been told about Prime Minister Blair's plans to reform the NHS. "*Just who does he think he is?*" one of them expostulates. The consequences of joining in a national tax funded health system seemed to be hitting him and his colleagues for the first time more than 50 years after it had happened.

These feelings can lead to alienation from the NHS and to some doctors wanting to opt out of decision making roles, leaving everything to others, so that they can "*just carry on being a doctor*". This is very problematic given both doctors' natural leadership roles in most situations and the impact their decisions make on resources and the activities of others. There have been many attempts in recent years to engage doctors more in formal leadership and management roles, some more successful than others. In 2011 Andrew Lansley, the current Secretary of State, is once again trying to draw GPs in particular into such a role – and in doing so address one part of the 1948 compromise which allowed GPs to remain semi-detached from the rest of the NHS.

Meanwhile other groups and nurses in particular, have been going from strength to strength in taking on new roles and spreading their influence. Looking beyond the UK and other high income countries it is clear that nurses, not always defined as precisely or in the same way as in the UK, are the prime providers of care to billions.

This takes us to the second aspect about health workers: how they have become more professional and professionalised throughout the last century. The growing competence and capability and the adherence to standards and respect for evidence are all enormously welcome. The accompanying growth in power of the professions and their professional bodies is a mixed blessing. In some ways it drives standards but in others it secures advantages for their members through straight trade union bargaining power which may not be in the interest of the wider public as both patients and ultimate payers.

All professions have their positive and negative aspects. On the one hand professions promise to open careers to talent but on the other are monopolistic and self centred.[13]

These descriptions draw attention to the power of the professions, especially doctors, and to the way that they can align with other powerful interests in commerce and academia to set the agenda for healthcare and secure benefits for themselves. There is an extensive literature about the American so-called *medico-*

industrial complex, first described in 1971, which highlights the way that the big commercial businesses of pharmaceuticals and medical supplies, the massive healthcare institutions, the universities and even government can combine to treat healthcare as just another for-profit business with the same motivations and behaviours as any other.[14] Many authors have described the problems of overuse of tests and procedures, fragmentation of services and overemphasis on technological solutions which can result from this.[15] It is very easy for doctors, with all their knowledge and authority to encourage patients to spend more on another test, another procedure or another treatment. This is a market failure which is easily exploited by the unscrupulous.

The situation in the UK is rather different because most health care is funded by the NHS and many of the same incentives don't apply. However, there seems little doubt that pharmaceutical companies have, in the past at least, sought to influence doctors to use their products by offering incentives to doctors to learn more about them. Processes have now been tightened up and controls introduced. I recall being told that almost all the orthopaedic surgeons in one part of the country had been taught to ski by the same medical products company which had organised orthopaedic training courses in European resorts. I suppose a ski slope is a good place to be learning about fractures and torn tendons. Few people who worked in the NHS in the 1990s would be surprised by this story.

The most important issue here is that this alignment of the interests of the medical professions and some commercial enterprises tends to keep the focus on treatment rather than on prevention. It reinforces a view of healthcare as being about the use of increasingly high tech solutions in hospitals to address complex problems and ignores the many things which in reality have a bigger impact on health.

It sets an agenda that is about doctors, hospitals and ever more sophisticated treatments carried out by specialists. The trouble is that we need one that is about prevention, healthy lifestyles, low-tech non-intrusive treatments in community settings which are carried out by a range of different people including the patient.

Patients and professionals

The third and perhaps the biggest change in recent years is in the way in which the relationships between professionals and patients have changed and are still changing. People, as John Reid observed, are not willing to accept the norms of the NHS of 1948 in 2000. The more educated and emancipated patients of today are no longer willing to treat doctors, nurses and other health workers with the same level of deference as they did 50 years ago. The elite are being challenged in healthcare as in every other aspect of life. Moreover, patient involvement in care is now seen to be clinically beneficial.

This relationship was severely tested even as the NHS Plan was being developed and implemented by a series of investigations and inquiries that shook and are still shaking the NHS. In 1998 a public inquiry was set up under the Chairmanship of Sir Ian Kennedy to review the large number of deaths of small children at the Bristol Royal Infirmary between 1984 and 1995 whilst undergoing or as a result of cardiac surgery.

Three short extracts from its 2001 final report illustrate the Inquiry's findings:

> *"The story of the paediatric cardiac surgical service in Bristol is not an account of bad people. Nor is it an account of people who did not care, nor of people who wilfully harmed patients."*

> *"It is an account of a hospital where there was a 'club culture'; an imbalance of power, with too much control in the hands of a few individuals."*

> *"The NHS must root out unsafe practices. It must remove barriers to safe care. In particular, it must promote openness and the preparedness to acknowledge errors and to learn lessons. Healthcare professionals should have a duty of candour to patients."*[16]

These three extracts reinforce some of the themes in this chapter about systems, attitudes and power and raise questions about the accountability not just of doctors but of the whole NHS. A second Inquiry was set up when it was discovered during the course of the Bristol Inquiry that organs and tissue from children had been retained for medical research apparently without informing parents or seeking their permission.

The Royal Liverpool Children's Hospital Inquiry reported in January 2001 only months after publication of the NHS Plan. Whilst it recognised that the worst problems were due to one individual, it also noted that the practice was widespread:

> *"The practice we have described seems to have been of general application. The medical justification is a manifestation of the paternalistic approach, namely the policy of restricting the freedom and responsibility of parents in their supposed best interests. In mitigation, it is stated that the heart collection has served to reduce the mortality rate following cardiac surgery for some serious conditions and malformations from 33% to 3%. This benefit cannot be ignored, but it is no justification for ignoring the parents' rights."*[17]

It showed how far NHS and medical practice had become separated from public opinion. Such behaviour may have been reasonable in 1948 but to a 21st century public it was scandalous. Power had shifted, deference was disappearing.

25

I know that many pathologists and other doctors found this extremely troubling. They were, as they pointed out, only collecting materials for the public good. They were doing something which they saw as being their duty. The public's view, however, was that they had got it the wrong way round. The first priority was to respect the family's decision making and then work out how to get material for research rather than give priority to the research. The Human Tissue Act 2004 redressed the balance although, in the view of many clinicians, it has now made it too difficult to collect such materials for research.

The Shipman Inquiry opened in 2000 to investigate how a GP had been able to murder 250 or more patients without detection by colleagues or anyone within the NHS. This was very different to Bristol and Liverpool. No one believed that Shipman was anything but a ghastly exception. The issue was why he had gone undetected so long: why hadn't colleagues had suspicions, why wasn't the exceptional use of morphine picked up and why wasn't the pattern of deaths noticed? As NHS Chief Executive I recall giving evidence to the Inquiry and agonising over how we could be absolutely certain that no one could ever do this again. Dame Janet Smith who led the Inquiry recommended new processes and systems in her 2005 report to try to ensure this. She also criticised the role of the General Medical Council (GMC) which registered doctors for being too supportive of them:

> "I have concluded that, in approaching such cases as it did, the GMC focussed too much on the interests of the doctors and not sufficiently on the public interest and the need for patients to be protected from drug abusing doctors."[18]

These three inquiries specifically involved doctors. However, in 2011 we are awaiting the final deliberations of the Public Inquiry into events at Mid Staffordshire NHS Foundation Trust.[19]

Anyone reading the evidence to the Inquiry will be shocked by the behaviour and seemingly casual neglect shown by some members of staff that was not checked by others. It is shaming for all of us who were involved in the NHS at the time. Here, as with the Shipman Inquiry, the biggest questions seem to be why didn't people outside the Trust know what was going on, why wasn't it stopped and how far did national policies, which I of course promoted at the start of the period covered, contribute to the local tragedy?

Whatever the Inquiry concludes, the analysis to date demonstrates the importance of promoting patient and public perceptions as a counter balance to the power of the professions and the NHS institutions that run the NHS. In Mid Staffordshire as in Bristol the Inquiries were held primarily because of the actions of patients' groups. It took too long but eventually their concerns were heard.

New arrangements are needed which put patients and citizens at the heart of the NHS social contract.

Health and society: patients and citizens

The development of patient and public power and the engagement of patients in their own care and in designing new service models will undoubtedly be amongst the most important themes in healthcare over the next few years. They are the only forces strong enough in the end to overcome the inertia and vested interests of those seeking to maintain the status quo.

I believe that this will herald a fundamental change in how we think about health and healthcare in the future and how we judge success or failure. Ultimately, as I will argue, healthcare is about helping people live lives they have reason to value. It is about individual's perceptions and judgements.

What people believe about themselves and their health and how much faith they have in health professionals all affect what health care they are willing to accept and what professionals can do. The experience of health workers trying to vaccinate populations shows this very clearly. Around 15% of London parents refused the MMR vaccination for their children in the early years of this century because they were led to believe that it might cause autism. As a result measles is back in London and is killing children. There are many other similar examples which are very difficult to counter.[20]

A study in Ethiopia shows that even when healthcare is available in a low income country people choose whether to use it based on their own assessment of how ill they are, whether they think the services available will help them and how difficult it is reach them.[21] Patients make their own trade-offs. We all do – as the millions of unfinished courses of medicine in our bathroom cupboards, as well as the millions of unfilled prescription scripts in countries like the US where patients pay directly for their medicine, testify.

Our ambivalent attitudes to the health advice given to us by health professionals about what to eat and drink, how much exercise we need and how to have sex as well as our growing consumption of "health products" all reinforce the point about our decision making. The increasing use of biological diagnostics to predict the chances of future illness brings with it an even greater space for individual trade-offs as we each choose what to believe and whether an increased risk of coronary heart disease of X% justifies our taking evasive action.

Research shows that when it comes to many of these decisions it is our peers and friends rather than health professionals who often influence our choices and behaviours.[22]

The Commission on the Social Determinants of Health has demonstrated clearly that social issues matter in other perhaps more fundamental ways too.[23] Our health is in large part determined by our position in society, our socio-economic status and our inclusion or exclusion in society. It is not just about income – although income is the factor most closely correlated with health – but also about all the things that are often related to income such as education, housing, clean environments, safety and greater self worth and fulfilment. These are averages of course; individuals can and do improve or ruin their own health by their actions. Money may not bring health any more than it brings happiness but it can certainly help.

A boy born in affluent parts of southern England today has a life expectancy 10 years greater than one born in a poor part of the north. The pattern is repeated around the world. The social gradient from the richest and most successful in a society to the poorest and least successful matches the health gradient from healthiest and longest lived to the sickest and shortest lived.

In the face of all this evidence of the important impacts that society has on health it is perhaps surprising that we almost always begin our thinking about health in terms of health professionals and healthcare systems. We deal with doctors and hospitals and patients not health and citizens. In reality of course the drama of acute illness and emergencies and the charisma and shaman-like properties of our healers easily claim the attention. We need to work hard to reverse this and start where we are – with our lives and our society – and then accommodate the technical knowledge and the professional within our thinking.

Society is changing and with it the scope for health improvement and the risks to health change too. Our understanding of health and disease is also developing fast. Together these wider environmental changes mean that Governments and those charged with improving health and running health systems need to be constantly adapting their policies and practices.

Global trends

The reforms in the English NHS took place in a fast changing world where four major global trends were already beginning to have an effect on health and healthcare.

There have been remarkable improvements in health over the last century. Life expectancy for a man in the UK has increased by 30 years in a century. Globally, life expectancy has more than doubled in a century, in large part due to improvements in infant and child mortality. Better social and environmental conditions, increased affluence and better education have been the main contributors but, of course, better health care, better medication and better health workers have played their part.

It is a great success story but conditions have changed and health policies and services designed for one set of problems are now faced with another. Policies, services and practices need to be re-designed as a result.

The first trend is that the diseases we suffer from have changed. We no longer suffer and die from the same mix of causes. A century ago in the UK and other high income countries we were faced with many more infectious diseases, more trauma and more acute conditions. Now we have more cancer, more non-communicable diseases and a need for longer term rather than so much acute care.[24] Many of our diseases today are linked to life style and behaviour. Our hospital and doctor centred services simply aren't well geared to deal with them.

Low and middle income countries still have high levels of infectious or communicable diseases, most notably malaria, HIV/AIDS and TB but are also beginning to be affected by the same epidemic of non-communicable diseases. South Africa, for example, faces the four epidemics of communicable diseases, non-communicable diseases, maternal mortality and physical trauma.[25] In time, and as other improvements are made, non-communicable diseases will come to dominate.

The second trend is the way that patients and the public have changed. They are no longer willing simply to do as the doctor or nurse tells them. Moreover, the prevention and treatment of many of their diseases and conditions relies heavily on their involvement. They, or I should say we, also want to be treated personally as the individuals we are.

The third global trend is that science and technology are developing very fast. Any casual observer will know how much healthcare has changed in the last few years with, to take only a few examples, the introduction of keyhole surgery, the development of new radiological equipment and techniques which allow clinicians to unblock arteries and the various scopes which permit them see what is going on inside our bodies without having to cut us open to do so.

What is rarely seen is the human resources and facilities issues that these changes raise. There is a need for re-training of people. This can sometimes be resisted by the recipients. I recall a surgeon in the late 80s telling me that day surgery would never catch on because the patients wouldn't like it and therefore he didn't need to change his practice. It was wishful thinking on his part. There can be turf wars between for example the interventional radiologists and cardiologists on the one side and the surgeons on the other. In many cases the surgeons can see part of their traditional work disappearing into the Cath Labs and the CT, MRI and more advanced scanners which are operated by other people. There will almost certainly be a need for changes in facilities.

This sort of disruption will become more pronounced in the future as the new biology combines with information and communications technology to make patient monitoring at home, disease prediction and prevention, treatments in the community and much more, the norm rather than the exception. Whole hospital outpatient departments and the painstakingly learned skills of groups of health workers will disappear.

This disruption also raises some profound questions which need to be addressed both globally and within any health system about whether all such new scientific and technological invention is always beneficial, whether such inventiveness is directed to the right targets – to prevention rather than treatment, for example –

and about whether it is going to be available to benefit everyone. There are no easy answers.

The fourth disruption can sometimes be overlooked. The world is now far more interdependent in health terms than it has ever been. The processes of globalisation are affecting health as much as anything else. The area where we see this most clearly is in the transmission of disease. We are all potentially at risk from the same new and old communicable diseases and are concerned about pandemics that can rapidly become global. Some of the new diseases will arise in the poorest parts of the world where, without adequate surveillance and health services, they may well get a foothold and be able to spread worldwide. We share vulnerability. It is in our own self-interest to help create functioning health systems everywhere as a front line of defence against disease.

Climate change and other environmental issues cross boundaries – rain in the Himalayas affects Bangladesh, radioactive pollution in Russia affects Europe, mercury in fish stocks affects global markets – and need cross-boundary action.

We also share a dependence on the same groups of health workers who have become the first truly global professions able to work almost anywhere they choose. We share the same drugs and, often, treatment methodologies and knowledge. None of these, however, are shared equally around the world. The worst large scale example of this inequity is the way that Sub Saharan Africa with about 10% of the world's population and 25% of the world's burden of disease has only 3% of the world's health resources and about 1.5% of the world's supply of health workers to deal with it.[26]

I have described the current situation in another book – *Turning the World Upside Down – the search for global health in the 21st century* – as an unfair health trade.[27] Rich countries import trained health workers from poorer ones and in exchange export their ideas and ideologies about health and healthcare, whether they work or not. What would it be like, I ask, if we turned this upside down and exported some of the health workers from richer countries to poorer ones and imported some of their ideas and experiences about healthcare?

Migration to the UK, primarily from Sub Saharan Africa and South East Asia, has been a very important issue with the UK benefiting greatly from this transfer of personnel and their skills and energies. During the period covered by this book the UK responded by increasing its own training levels and became broadly self-sufficient by 2006, closing the doors on many would be migrants and, much more controversially, on some already in the country. It was one of many human resources reforms introduced in the English NHS during this period.

I also argued in that book that richer countries have a great deal that they can learn about improving health and health services from poorer ones. Without our resources, our historical baggage and our vested interests they can, and many do, innovate much more freely. Knowledge transfer is not all from the rich and powerful to the poor and weak but is, rather, a two way process. It is a simple argument that will surely become commonplace over the next decade as we in Europe and North America learn more about what is happening, to take the obvious example, in India.

Further global aspects which as yet do not affect the NHS to any extent but may be important in years to come are international regulation, trade and competition law. Europe is already encroaching on the freedoms the UK has to manage its health services and in the longer term competition law may directly challenge the rights of local people and of GPs to establish and run their own services free from competition.

Finally, the global recession and the UK's financial position will influence what is possible. The optimistic and expansionist early years of the century have been replaced by austerity and reductions in public spending.

There seems to be a simple choice about whether financial restrictions lead the NHS and other systems to limit their provision and look for co-payments from patients or, on the other hand, choose to re-design their services and systems to meet the financial restraints. The financial situation is likely to force the issue one way or the other.

If we get it right we will not only save the NHS as a system that provides care for everyone but also put it on a sustainable and strong footing for the future.

Conclusions and key points

1. By 1999 the NHS had multiple problems and was in decline. Poor systems, lack of resources, low morale and an absence of overall direction all contributed to inadequate clinical results and unsatisfactory care for patients.

2. The overall framework of the NHS with its emphasis on primary care and equity was robust. However, in order to survive the NHS needed a clear direction, greater unity of purpose, new energy and resources and a radical overhaul of systems, incentives and organisation. Incremental changes would not do. This required a massive reform programme and a major act of political will.

3. Health is always a political issue and the provision of healthcare is very closely related to how people see the world and what aspirations they have for their society. It can't be treated in isolation from other social and economic policies. Health reform in the UK was part of wider efforts to re-define and re-shape the 50 year old Welfare State.

4. There are many different perspectives in healthcare and many powerful interests. The strength of these provider and staff interests can serve patients and the public well but they can also distort priorities and lead to a closed and patronising culture which doesn't listen to their needs or value their views.

5. There have been three broad shifts in power over the years with doctors giving up some power to other groups, the professions becoming more closed and powerful, and the public becoming more demanding. These all shaped the reforms.

6. New ways are needed to promote patients and citizens as a counter balance to the power of the professions and other interests and to engage them more fully in their own care and in the design of services.

7. Four major global trends affect planning and policy:
   a. Non-communicable diseases and long term conditions are now the main causes of illness and death and the biggest consumers of healthcare resources. Community and people based services are needed for these diseases to replace the hospital and doctor based services which were required 50 years ago.
   b. Patients and the public are becoming both more assertive and more important in the prevention, cure and management of disease.
   c. Technology and science are providing new solutions which require new services to be designed and make old ways of working redundant.
   d. The world is becoming ever more interdependent in health terms with the global spread of diseases, reliance on the same resources and staff and the need to align policies regionally and globally.

8. The financial situation is likely to force the choice about whether the NHS restricts the services available or takes the harder option of changing the way it provides services and releases costs from the old infrastructure and traditional practices.

References

1. OECD Health data 2010.
2. Office of Health Economics: *Compendium of Health Statistics*; 2006.
3. Department of Health: *The NHS Plan – a plan for investment, a plan for reform*; Cmd 4818-1, The Stationary Office, 2000 p 31.
4. Wanless D (2002) *Our future health: taking a long-term view*; HM Treasury.

5. The Commonwealth Fund (2006) *Why not the best?*: Figure 11 p 26.
6. The National Health Service Act 1946.
7. Beveridge Report: the Report of the Inter-Departmental Committee on Social Insurance and Allied Services 1942.
8. Timmins N (1995) *The Five Giants – a biography of the Welfare State*. Harper Collins.
9. *Aneurin Bevan on the National Health Service*; The Wellcome Unit for the History of Medicine, Oxford 1991.
10. Reid TR (2009) *The Healing of America: a global quest for better, cheaper and fairer healthcare*, Penguin Press.
11. Sir Roy Griffiths (1983) Griffiths Report – *NHS Management Inquiry*. Department of Health.
12. Moss-Kanter R (2011) *Why innovation is so hard to do in healthcare and how to do it anyway*; Blog from Harvard Business Review and Harvard University *Advanced Leadership Initiative*; 22 Feb.
13. Menand L (2010) *The marketplace of ideas: reform and resistance in the American university*; New York, WW Norton and Company, pp 101–102
14. Ehrenreich B and Ehrenreich J (1971) *The American Health Empire*; Health-PAC.
15. Reman AS (1980) The new medical-industrial complex. *New England Journal of Medicine*, **303**: 963–70.
16. Bristol Royal Infirmary Inquiry: Synopsis paras 3–14; July 2001.
17. Royal Liverpool Children's Hospital Inquiry; Summary paragraph 13.
18. Shipman Inquiry 5th Report CM 6394 Dec 2004; paragraph 96.
19. Mid Staffordshire NHS Foundation Trust Inquiry Final Report February 2010.
20. Cooper LZ, Larson HJ, Katz SL (2008) Protecting public trust in immunization. *Paediatrics*, **122**: 1–5.
21. Petricca K, Mamo Y, Haileamlak A, Seid E, Parry E: *Barriers to effective follow up treatment of rheumatic heart disease in rural Ethiopia. A grounded theory analysis of the patient experience*; unpublished paper.
22. Leydon GM, Bynoe-Sutherland J, Coleman MP (2003) The journey towards a cancer diagnosis: the experiences of people with cancer, their family and carers. *Eur Journal of Cancer Care (Engl)*, **12**(4): 317–26.
23. World Health Organisation (2008) *Closing the gap in a generation: Health equity through action on the social determinants of health*; Commission on Social Determinants of Health.
24. Hicks J, Allen G (1999) *Causes of death in England and Wales 1880-1997; from A Century of change: trends in UK statistics since 1900*; House of Commons Library research paper 99/111.
25. Mayosi BM, Flisher AJ, Lalloo UG, Sitas F, Tollman SM, Bradshaw D (2009) The burden of non-communicable diseases in South Africa. *The Lancet*, **374** (9693): 934–47.
26. Crisp N (2010) *Turning the World Upside Down – the search for global health in the 21st century*; RSM Press, p 30.
27. Ibid.

Chapter 3

The NHS Plan – overview of the story

The story opens with a round of applause.

Alan Milburn, the Secretary of State for Health, was waiting to announce the launch of the NHS Plan in the House of Commons. Many of the great and good of UK healthcare were watching him on television, seated around the long meeting table in his Whitehall office together with his aides and a cluster of civil servants. As the Secretary of State rose to speak, Sir George Alberti, President of the Royal College of Physicians and one of the most senior doctors in the land, started to slap the table with his hand. The action was taken up by others and as Milburn started speaking there was a thundering tribute of hands clapping together in time on the table.

It was spring 2000. The Prime Minister had said that the UK should increase spending on the NHS up to the European average level. It was confirmed in the Budget. George and other senior figures had met with the Prime Minister and the Chancellor. There had been many behind the scenes discussions, announcements in Parliament and everything was now falling into place.

Over the next few weeks a collection of some 135 people – patients, professionals, politicians, advisers and civil servants – would work in teams to draw up plans to modernise the NHS. The resulting NHS Plan which brought together their work set out a blueprint for the next 10 years.[1] It was published on 1 July just four days before the 52nd anniversary of the founding of the NHS.

It was a glorious moment of triumph not just for Milburn but for the others in the room, many of whom as leaders of nursing, medical and other organisations had argued and lobbied for this and would put themselves on the line and, quite literally, sign up to the values incorporated in the NHS Plan. It was an excellent start to the reforms: an encouraging and uplifting prologue, with a plan, money and a unified leadership. Almost anyone might have joined in the applause that that day.

I wasn't in the room myself and hadn't been part of the process but it would determine my life for the next six years. Later that year I was appointed to lead the implementation of the Plan and given unprecedented authority as Chief Executive of the NHS and Permanent Secretary of the Department of Health.

The NHS Plan – subtitled *a plan for investment, a plan for reform* – is an optimistic, wide ranging and very ambitious document. It confidently sets out a 10 year programme of improvement which is designed to "*… give people a service fit for the 21st century. A service designed around the patient.*"[2]

> ### Box 3.1 The NHS Plan[3]
>
> *Our vision: a health service designed around the patient*
> - **Preventive care** ... routine screening will be extended ... at the forefront of assessing new medicines ... maintain registers ... check that older people living alone are all right ... NHSplus an occupational health service
> - **Self care** ... NHS Direct 24/7 phone line and internet ... digital TV
> - **Primary care** ... one stop shop for access and service via NHS Direct ... round the clock care for minor ailments and accidents provided locally ... electronic patient records ... teams working in multi-purpose premises
> - **Hospital care** ... appointments pre-booked ... tests and diagnosis on same day ... ¾ of operations as day cases ... traditional waiting list will disappear ... diagnosis and treatment centres ... referral to specialist centres ... a new generation of state of the art hospitals ... "modern matrons" ... personal TVs ... patient advocates
> - **Intermediate care** ... new services ... a bridge between hospital and home ... rapid response and hospital at home ... new technology
> - **Quality of care** ... every unit will publish an annual prospectus on standards, performance and the views of patients ... funding dependent on patient views ... national standards for major conditions ... standard protocols ... independent inspection.

It was truly comprehensive and Box 3.1, taken from the section on vision, gives a hint of the extraordinary range and detail of the document. The Plan really acted as a focus for bringing together all the ideas, hopes and aspirations of the people involved in the process and of many others outside it. It was what they all wanted the NHS to become as it dragged itself up from the depression and despondency of the 80s and 90s.

The full document sets out even more goals and more than 200 targets for the NHS to achieve. They included increases in inputs as well as improvements in services and health outcomes. There were targets to recruit 10,000 more doctors and 30,000 more nurses. There were targets for reducing waiting times and for opening new services. There were targets for reduction in premature deaths from cancer and coronary heart disease and for reduction in suicides. There were targets for the NHS and for Social Services and for the two to achieve together.

My father, with long experience in industry, read the Plan, noted all the targets and recalled that the Labour Party Manifesto for the 1987 election had been described as the longest suicide note in history. This he told me was the longest suicide note ever written for a Chief Executive in history.

Despite this dampener, I accepted the job with great enthusiasm when it was offered to me.

Overview

This chapter gives an overview of the implementation of the Plan during the time I was Chief Executive between 2000 and 2006 and a brief outline of the final years up to 2010.

It provides rather more detail on the start up phase and the mobilisation of people and resources. The later stages when delivery actually started to happen and when reforms started to bite are covered in greater depth in the following four chapters. Each of these concentrates on one of the four domains of reform – service re-design, system reform, restructuring the workforce and improving the use of knowledge, science and technology in the NHS.

Appendix 3 provides a brief chronology of significant events during this period within a longer time line of all the reforms since 1985.

Building the will and creating the Plan

The creation of the NHS Plan was preceded by increased public dissatisfaction with the state of the NHS, which had been heightened by its perceived failure to deal with flu and other "winter pressures" at the beginning of the year, and political dissatisfaction with slow improvement. Not for the first time in the NHS's history, something needed to be done. The Prime Minister responded to the problems in January 2000 during a television interview by promising to increase NHS spending to the European average. His promise was converted into a commitment to specific budgetary increases in March. Something would be done.

The Secretary of State for Health, Alan Milburn, and his advisers took up the challenge with vigour and set about creating a plan to spend the money well and achieve real improvement. They, wisely, decided on a process which would engage stakeholders whilst building up a detailed plan.

They did this in two main ways. Firstly, they ran two consultations, one for the public and one for staff, to ask what people saw as the priorities for improvement and, secondly, they brought together the 135 people mentioned earlier and gave them a very tight timetable to shape the plans in five areas – the five "P's" of partnership; performance; professions and the wider NHS workforce; patient care; and prevention. They created a *Modernisation Action Team* led by a Minister in each of these areas and one that dealt with cross-cutting issues. They had four months to report with a detailed assessment of the current position and a radical path forward.

This process was led politically, but it was also very well managed. Many of the leading figures in health were easily persuaded to join the effort. Here was an activist Secretary of State with the support of the Prime Minister – and the promise of money – asking them to join in planning improvement. There was no question but that they had to be part of it. Although this work took place outside the normal management process the then NHS Chief Executive, Sir Alan Langlands identified a young manager to be the project manager and draw all the themes together into a coherent plan and made sure that others from the Department were available to help each group and coordinate the work.

More than 10 years later Mike Deegan, the young project manager who is now a successful Chief Executive of a major Teaching Hospital Foundation Trust, told me: "*At times the tight deadline meant that the process felt like a roller coaster ride; but ministerial leadership and the timescale gave the process real momentum and dynamism.*"

It proved to be very successful. The Secretary of State had bought in many of the key stakeholders and secured some public legitimacy from the surveys; but he had also retained the ability in the end to shape and edit the final plan in private with his advisers. The resulting NHS Plan was very definitely his plan.

As importantly, it was the Prime Minister's plan. It was not, initially at least, the Treasury's plan. Whilst the NHS Plan was very concerned with healthcare and service delivery the Treasury's and the Chancellor's instincts were much more orientated towards health and promoting policies for health promotion, healthy living and the prevention of disease. These, they believed with some reason, were not only more cost effective but more effective in the long run.

The public's priority, however – and therefore the government's imperative – was the immediacy of service provision not the slow burn of health improvement. The Government which three years before had said there was 24 hours to save the NHS hadn't made good progress with it. Health was high profile and the Government was very vulnerable to any failure here. Healthcare and service provision had to take precedence, with health and prevention coming later. It is a tension which is familiar to any health policy maker or planner and which is the despair of any public health worker.

The problem was simple: if you didn't tackle the immediate problems that people were worried about you wouldn't be trusted – or granted the time – to take on the others. Later on, as we shall see, we benefited from the "waiting list dividend". We had managed to reduce the waiting lists and so had created the space to take on the wider and longer term health issues.

There was, as always with this Government, tension between the Treasury and Number 10 but, thanks to many behind the scenes negotiations, mostly as hidden from me as from the public, the Plan and its funding were brought together and cross-Government support established. Extra funding had been granted to the NHS in the April 2000 Budget shortly after the Prime Minister's commitment but the Treasury had not been fully bought in. They did their own review as we shall see in the next section and it was not till April 2002 that the funding needed to implement the Plan fully was in place.

It was smart politics. The Secretary of State had done extremely well to get Prime Minister, Chancellor and stakeholders lined up – and to do so very quickly in a few fevered months of activity. There could hardly have been a better or more auspicious context for the NHS Plan. The content itself, however, had some significant flaws and hid some serious problems in amongst its great strengths and the passion and energy with which it was launched. Two problems stand out.

The first was that the consultation surveys, although achieving high numbers of returns with 152,000 public and 58,000 staff respondents, produced results that were couched in such general terms that they could be interpreted in many different ways. People wanted "*more, better paid staff*", "*more prevention*", "*care centred on patients*" and "*improvements in local hospitals and surgeries*".[4]

There was overlap between patient and staff views but there were some interesting differences. The most obvious of which was the public demand for cleaner hospitals – "*Cleanliness, cleanliness, cleanliness – employ more cleaners in hospital*"[5] – whilst staff make no mention of this. It was a clear signal that wasn't picked up at the time and a topic which would come back to haunt us.

The second was that the Plan failed to resolve one of the dilemmas facing any attempt to improve a national health system: how to make sure your plan is implemented as you want it whilst allowing local leaders to make decisions about what is most needed in their areas and what will work most effectively there. This national versus local tension was a continuing theme throughout the period.

The Plan says at many points that it will be implemented through the efforts of local people and that "*a key message arising from the consultation with the NHS in formulating this Plan was that it needs a small focussed set of targets to drive change. Too many targets simply overwhelm the service.*"[6]

It goes on in the same passage to identify a list of 13 "*must do targets*" which are reproduced in Appendix 4. They are pretty extensive in their own right. However, only 10 pages earlier and throughout much of the document the Plan includes many far more detailed targets. It says, for example, in relation to mental health that "*by 2003 all 20,000 people estimated to need assertive outreach will be receiving these services*" and that "*by 2004, services will be designed to ensure that there are women-only day centres in every health authority compared with only a handful at present.*"[7]

The stated intentions were worthy but the prescription threatened to overwhelm the NHS – even if we did have 10 years to deliver all these targets.

Despite these serious reservations, there was no doubt that Alan Milburn had achieved in 2000 what most health ministers could only dream of. Now all he – and subsequently I – had to worry about was the sniping from other Departments which had been less successful in gaining priority and resources. There was, of course, also the small matter of implementation and delivery.

Funding

The NHS was given a 6.1% annual increase for four years in the 2000 but more was needed to reach the European average which the Prime Minister had specified as his target level.

The Chancellor re-took control of the NHS budget by setting up his own review of health expenditure. He invited the former National Westminster Bank Chief Executive, Derek Wanless, to determine the likely costs of the health service over the next 20 years. Wanless undertook this task by looking at overall health need, making comparisons with other countries and, using diabetes as the example, working out what likely costs might be.

It was a very important and influential piece of work both because it secured the money that the NHS needed but also because, for the first time, a thorough bottom up approach was taken to healthcare costs. Its analysis has continuing relevance today.

Wanless's report, *Securing Our Future Health: Taking a Long-Term View, April 2002* described three scenarios – "*solid progress*", where there was some change in public behaviour and some improvement in the use of technology and in outcomes; "*slow uptake*" where there was no change in behaviour, low uptake of technology and poor results generally; and a "*fully engaged*" scenario where patients took much more control of their own health, there was good use of technology and good approaches to disease prevention.[8] These are described in Box 3.2.

Box 3.2 Summary of the three scenarios in the Wanless Review[9]

The resources required to deliver a high quality service will depend on the health needs and demands of the population, technological developments, workforce issues and productivity. As there is uncertainty around how these additional cost drivers will change, the Review has built up three scenarios:

- *Solid progress* – people become more engaged in relation to their health: life expectancy rises considerably, health status improves and people have confidence in the primary care system and use it more appropriately. The health service is responsive with high rates of technology uptake and a more efficient use of resources;

- *Slow uptake* – there is no change in the level of public engagement: life expectancy rises by the lowest amount in all three scenarios and the health status of the population is constant or deteriorates. The health service is relatively unresponsive with low rates of technology uptake and low productivity; and

- *Fully engaged* – levels of public engagement in relation to their health are high: life expectancy increases go beyond current forecasts, health status improves dramatically and people are confident in the health system and demand high quality care. The health service is responsive with high rates of technology uptake, particularly in relation to disease prevention. Use of resources is more efficient.

The Review's assumptions about pay, prices and the configuration of the workforce are common across all scenarios.

The emphasis on prevention and "full engagement" was not new but the consolidation and bringing together of the evidence in this way was. It fitted far better with a Treasury approach to prevention rather than a Number 10 one to service provision. It was Number 10, however, that prevailed and we concentrated on service provision rather than *full engagement* in the years that followed. Still today we have not put anything like the same level of energy and resources into prevention as we have into treatment.

Wanless provided a range of likely cost based on the 3 scenarios at the time of the Budget in April 2002 which showed that the NHS needed an increase of up to 7.3% in real terms for five years to "catch up" on the lost investment over recent years and move expenditure from an estimated 7.7% of GDP in 2002/03 to an estimated 9.5% by 2007/08. He proposed that it should rise more slowly thereafter but would still need to be between 10.6% and 12.5% of GDP by 2022/23 to maintain the progress.[10] These figures almost precisely matched our Departmental ones. Number 10, the Treasury and the Department of Health had worked together well. We had full cross Government buy-in.

Mobilisation

As Chief Executive I inherited an outline of an implementation strategy. The NHS Plan stated that a Modernisation Board would be created from amongst some of the stakeholders to oversee the whole process; the new NHS Chief Executive would be appointed; the Modernisation Board would agree and publish a detailed implementation programme in the autumn; more money would be made available immediately to increase the number of heart operations and make a good start on improvements; and, in a real departure for government, Health Authorities would be given three year budgets from 2001, allowing them to plan more securely.[11]

These were all good measures but were in truth only a preliminary sketch of what was needed. This next phase, which lasted throughout 2001, was about mobilising the people and the resources to implement the Plan. Reality is always far messier than the theory and this period was no exception and it took some time to find and put in place an effective implementation strategy.

I started with what I was given. The Modernisation Board was a political confection which had no executive responsibilities. It brought together more than 30 of the key figures in English healthcare – a mixture of clinicians, patients' group leaders, managers and policy makers – and was chaired jointly by the Secretary of State and the Chief Executive. It never had a defined and formal role but was really an advisory group of stakeholders who were able, mostly rather gently, to challenge the Secretary of State and Chief Executive and to receive updates from them.

It was very effective as a means of getting messages out to the NHS and its partners and to the media. It kept us in touch with some of the key strands of opinion – it contained some very impressive leaders – and allowed us to influence them and them to influence us. It was another very smart element in the management of change and engagement of stakeholders that had begun with the Modernisation Action Teams and was ably supported by Sian Jarvis, who became Director of Communications in July 2001, and Chris Ham and others in the Department's Strategy Unit.

Like all informal and advisory arrangements which have no authority or status of their own its role was very dependent on personalities and relationships. It lasted throughout Alan Milburn's time as Secretary of State, but really faded away to insignificance when John Reid became his successor in 2003 without any pre-existing knowledge of the people and with other ideas about delivery.

I was appointed as Chief Executive on 1st November 2000 with the brief to deliver the NHS Plan. For years, before it actually happened for the first time in 1985, Governments had wanted to appoint a powerful figure as Chief Executive of the NHS as a counter measure to the consensus management and drift that they saw in delivery.[12] Many of them had specifically wanted to appoint an experienced private sector figure, who knew about business and getting things done, and who would be, in their view, much more effective than public sector consensus builders.

In 2000 the Government once again looked for a private sector appointment but failed to find one. I suspect that, as on other occasions, many candidates were put off by the political nature of the job – and the sort of risks identified by my father – and others simply didn't have the experience to lead the biggest employer in the country with its many fold complexities.

On appointment I was surprised and rather intrigued to be introduced to a very high profile private sector leader with the suggestion that we might somehow work together. We met and discussed it but neither of us saw how it would work. It was a cordial meeting. We wished each other well and went off in our different directions.

I was appointed as both Chief Executive of the NHS in England and Permanent Secretary of the UK Department of Health. This was the first and last time that these roles were combined. It was designed to align the goals of NHS and Department and to allow the Chief Executive to exercise maximum authority. This approach had its detractors and was, in reality, full of tension; however, it did guarantee focus on the Government's goals and ensure that there was no inter-personal conflict at the top.

I also found that I had inherited 10 Task Forces which were set up in effect as successors to the Modernisation Action Teams to lead and oversee improvements in all the key areas of the Plan from access to mental health. I incorporated the Task Forces into the Implementation Plan which I presented to the Modernisation Board for agreement in December 2000, a month after my appointment.[13] It used a conceptual framework based on Kotter's work and set out plans for a guiding coalition of leaders; a clear vision; regular communication; quick wins; a broad base of activity; the mainstreaming of change and local ownership.[14]

The implementation plan offered a reasonable framework for action but didn't really address the question of how all this was going to be made to happen in reality. Who would act, how would they be held to account, how could we be sure that the changes would be enacted in every part of the country? The Task Forces, which initially attempted to issue guidance and monitor developments on every target everywhere, were a very bureaucratic tool and were quietly dropped over the next few months as we created a much more appropriate delivery and performance management structure.

Looking back the issue here was how to move from the inclusive processes needed in planning and building momentum to the accountability processes needed for delivery.

I had a wider inheritance, too, that reached back before the creation of the NHS Plan. There were many excellent people and a great deal to build on. I do not want to give the impression that everything was new or − as sometimes happens with new appointments − that all history started when I came on the scene. In particular there had been a lot of work done on quality and a new framework introduced, largely through the leadership of the new Chief Medical Officer, Sir Liam Donaldson.[15] This was probably the most significant achievement of the Labour years before the NHS Plan.

The quality framework brought together arrangements for standard setting, developing protocols and independent inspection as well as introducing a new duty of clinical governance for all NHS organisations.

The National Institute for Clinical Excellence (NICE) and the Commission for Health Improvement (CHI), the two bodies charged respectively with developing standards and assessing therapies for the NHS and for inspecting services and organisations, had been established in the last two years and were starting to operate. NICE and CHI and its successors performed very important functions in the re-shaping of the NHS and have perhaps even more important roles in today's more decentralised NHS.[16]

As important was the continuing work on creating National Service Frameworks (NSFs) which were precisely that: frameworks for major areas such as cancer or coronary heart disease which identified key targets and the most important levers for implementing them.

The Cancer Plan, the NSF prototype, contained 10 target areas from reducing smoking to increasing treatment levels and reinforced the role of networks of organisations involving primary, secondary and tertiary organisations in delivering high quality care.[17] Several more NSFs were published in the next few years, all of them led by National Clinical Directors, often known as Czars, and built up through a national consensus building process.

The Czars made an extremely important contribution to the NHS. They were high status clinicians who could influence their colleagues as well as the public – and politicians – and by accepting these roles they took on a personal responsibility for delivery. There were Czars involved in practically all the areas described in the next chapter where we saw great success in meeting targets and making significant improvements.

This quality framework was to survive throughout the NHS Plan reform years and Liam Donaldson was responsible for developing a number of new aspects and organisations, from a focus on patent safety incorporated in the National Patient Safety Agency to a mechanism for dealing with "problem doctors", the National Clinical Assessment Authority. It was probably more comprehensive than any quality framework in any other country in the world.

Organisation

Once appointed I had the opportunity to assemble a management team and make other key appointments both in the Department of Health and in the NHS. I had inherited structures which were geared towards other priorities and tasks and I needed to make some considerable rearrangement by bringing together, for example, people who had been working separately on health and social service issues. I also needed to make some key appointments of people who would take personal responsibility for particular target areas such as waiting times and primary care.

There were two main features in the new structures. The first was the introduction of greater accountability and a clearer management line. This involved making appointments in the Department and at the top of the NHS and streamlining the links between the Department and the front line. Neil McKay, a very experienced NHS manager, who had been acting NHS Chief Executive when I was appointed, took the lead in creating a delivery structure by appointing a number of strong managerial leaders from the NHS to work alongside the National Clinical Directors in all the main areas from cancer to access.

At the same time we set up the Modernisation Agency to help identify and spread best practice around the NHS. The Leadership Centre, created to develop clinical and managerial leaders throughout the NHS, was subsequently added to its responsibilities. Barbara Stocking, later the Director of Oxfam, was the first Modernisation Agency Chief Executive and brought together a good team of innovators in early 2001. The Delivery Directorate and the Modernisation Agency were to become the two essential arms of our delivery strategy for the next few years.

The organisational structure which linked the Chief Executive and the Department with front line hospitals and services also needed overhaul. In 1991, as a result of an earlier set of reforms, the Conservative Government had established the NHS Executive with headquarters in Leeds as an arm's length body to run the NHS. It hadn't worked as planned, largely because it was not established with any legal separation from the Department and senior staff spent most of their time in London where the Ministers were and where decisions were taken.[18]

When I was appointed as NHS Chief Executive I saw no operational reason to keep either the name NHS Executive or maintain the fiction that the NHS was headquartered in Leeds. I abolished the NHS Executive and moved the NHS Headquarters to London on the day of my appointment. I followed this up by creating a Management Board in London to replace the old NHS Executive Board. It was a sensible and pragmatic decision but naturally annoyed those members of the Department who had moved up to Leeds from London in the early 90s having been told that that was where the future was. A significant part of the Department remained and still remains in Leeds – and now that the Coalition Government has brought the process full circle and said that the NHS Commissioning Board will be based in Leeds – their future will be assured once again.

There was quite a complex structure between the headquarters of the NHS in the Department and the Trusts and PCTs where services were delivered with eight Regional Offices and 100 Health Authorities. This was rapidly slimmed down. Alan Milburn announced a reduction in the size of this structure in a speech in April 2001 at the launch of the Modernisation Agency. *Shifting the balance of power*, as the policy became known, was designed to give local organisations as much power as possible consistent with being part of a national service with national strategies and priorities.[19]

This reorganisation replaced the Regional Offices with four Directors of Health and Social Care. Each had the strategic and performance management oversight of the whole of health and social care in their area. We created 28 Strategic Health Authorities (SHAs) to replace the Health Authorities and take a more strategic and hands-off management role over a wider area. PCTs meanwhile would have the main management role working alongside Local Authorities to secure good local services for their populations.

We chose to make these changes as rapidly as possible so as not to lose momentum. Neil McKay led the transition process and we had the new arrangements operating in shadow form in the autumn of 2001 and given proper legal status the following April.

I had adopted a personal leadership style, which I discuss in much more detail in Chapter 9, whereby I concentrated on two things: results and inclusiveness. I knew that to achieve the results that were needed I had to find a way to engage as many of the leaders in the NHS as possible.

Accordingly from late 2001 I started to bring the SHA Chief Executives together on a monthly basis with my national Directors and the Czars as the "Top Team" of the NHS. It was a large group of about 50 but one which could be brought together regularly and permit me to develop a personal relationship with all my key leaders and for us together to develop a sense of becoming a real team. It became a crucial mechanism both for delivering results and for holding the organisation together as we went though turbulent times.

Getting the organisation right was crucial but re-organisation was disruptive and expensive with the loss of some very talented and experienced people and delay caused by some months of uncertainty as people were appointed – and disappointed – and new organisations formed.

Shifting the balance of power both decentralised and centralised at the same time. PCTs did gain more power but the clearer management lines also improved accountability and therefore allowed us to exercise more control from the centre. It gave the Chief Executive and Ministers the people and the levers to make change happen. It maintained the top down bottom up tension inherent in the Plan.

A slow start

Mobilisation and getting the right organisation took time and there was a lag before any results came through.

Given all the political will building and the difficult decisions that had been made it was not surprising that politicians wanted results and, in public relations terms, wanted, perhaps needed, them quickly. They had made all these promises to the electorate, where was the delivery? Ministers began to get impatient as 2001 wore on and there was no improvement.

Throughout this period the centre of Government comprising the Prime Minister's office, Number 10 Downing St, and the Treasury, Number 11 was also struggling to get the right organisational structure to drive improvements in public services. Following the 2001 election the Prime Minister wanted to increase the pace of public service reform and improvement. This led to the creation of a number of new units at Number 10 and the Treasury designed to aid improvements – dealing with efficiency, IT, public sector reform and much else.

Whilst this period lasted there was confusion, duplication and a certain amount of game playing as people struggled to identify clear roles and establish influence. Like us, they eventually settled down to a more consistent pattern of activity and behaviour with the establishment of the Prime Minister's Delivery Unit in June 2001. This coordinated most of the activity at the centre and continues in a modified form in the Treasury today.

These machinations complicated my and my colleagues' struggle to get the right organisation and to get delivery moving. So did events. We still had to manage all the issues that arise on a daily basis in an organisation as complex as the NHS.

The first two of four major scandals to hit the NHS had exploded to public notice just before this period. These were the deaths of children having heart surgery at the Bristol Royal Infirmary and the retention of patients' organs for research purposes without the permission of relatives at the Royal Liverpool Children's' Hospital at Alder Hey. These and the other two – the murder of many patients by GP Dr Shipman and, later, the mistreatment of patients at Mid Staffordshire NHS Foundation Trust – were to have a profound effect on relationships between the NHS and its professionals and the public and patients.

These scandals damaged confidence in the NHS and increased pressure for improvement. There was a great deal of scepticism about whether any improvement was possible and a large part of the media ran stories of individual cases of failure. They weren't hard to find. If we had a bad winter in 2001 it would only compound troubles.

It all added to the pressure on Ministers and on me and my team. The politicians were very conscious of the need to keep up the momentum and responded with a whole host of initiatives from appointing celebrity chefs to help improve hospital food, to mandating from the centre that small budgets should be given to all ward sisters for equipment and improvements. Some were very sensible, some were not. They maintained momentum of sorts in the media but, sometimes also distracted attention at the front line from the main task of securing the planned improvement.

I meanwhile found myself defending the indefensible in front of the Parliamentary Accounts Committee (PAC) when I was called to explain the management and, in some cases, manipulation of waiting list figures by a few Trust Chief Executives.[20] In the British system the PAC, a Committee of the House of Commons, scrutinises Government expenditure and holds the Permanent Secretary of each Department – the Accountable Officer for all the Departmental expenditure voted by Parliament – to account for spending and performance.

It was 14th January 2002, right at the end of this second phase and some Chief Executives and other senior staff had undoubtedly been massaging their waiting list figures to make them look better. I had to explain why several suspected culprits had resigned with a financial settlement from their employers rather than just being sacked. I did my best to explain that sometimes doing so was actually the cheapest and quickest option; but the Committee wanted exemplary punishment to encourage the others.

I ended up doing almost 30 of these hearings because of the high profile and the large expenditure increase for Health. It may still be a record for Permanent Secretaries; although not one I had ever coveted. It was no consolation either to know that film of that waiting list Inquiry was used for years afterwards as part of the training for civil servants attending their first PAC. It apparently showed the PAC at its most aggressive and a Permanent Secretary defending his Department well.

This was one of the first high profile arguments about figures and measurement which were to be such a regular theme over the next few years. The implementers of any improvement plan – in health or anywhere else – are vulnerable to accusations of fiddling figures and using the evidence that best suits the case. Equally, their opponents may do the same.

We consistently tried to counter this over the years by using auditors wherever we could – the Audit Commission were asked to do regular and unannounced spot-checks on waiting lists after the waiting list PAC. We also stuck consistently with the same definitions, for example about what constituted a waiting list or a hospital admission, which had been in force for many years. Nevertheless, the arguments about measurement continued and in some cases continue today.

The PAC hearing was a fitting end to this troubled period.

Delivery – at last

The winter of 2001 into 2002 brought the usual increase in emergencies, more frequent ambulance journeys and more A and E attendances, increased risk of flu, more people needing intensive care and difficulties in hospitals as they struggled to discharge elderly patients home or into nursing homes.

The NHS had greatly improved the management of these problems by 2001 and established a tightly run operation.[21] Trusts, PCTs and Local Authorities and Health Authorities prepared winter plans, flu vaccination was increased, extra intensive care beds were opened, and improved plans for providing back up from one hospital to another were in place. Centrally we required organisations to provide us with daily reports of any difficulties and we kept a close eye on problem areas.

It was a real command and control approach which was necessary at this stage of the NHS's history in order to improve services, enable the parts of the NHS to work better together and maintain public confidence. Our planning meant that we were now one step ahead of an aggressive media which was accustomed to find one problem with one patient somewhere in the NHS – an organisation which treated 1 million people every 36 hours, so problems weren't difficult to find – and use it to castigate the whole service. We now knew about any problems first.

The successful management of winter pressures gave us a degree of comfort and by the end of that financial year in March 2002 I was at last able to report some progress with waiting and other targets in my annual report.[22] They were pretty minimal improvements but the trend was now upwards and the next few years saw dramatic improvements in services and the expansion of staffing and facilities.

Neil McKay led a lot of the early delivery but decided to go back to the NHS and became the Chief Executive of the biggest hospital in the land, Leeds Teaching Hospitals NHS Trust. He was succeeded by John Bacon as Director General of Delivery initially on an acting basis in January 2003. He was ably supported by a group of performance managers, some focused on issues such as waiting and others on geographical areas. John effectively became my deputy in the NHS and his formidable team earned a reputation for toughness and for making sure that targets were delivered. By this time effective working relationships between managers, clinicians and politicians had been established in the Department and with Number 10 and there was a sense of common leadership and purpose.

Targets were hit, waiting lists fell, new hospitals were opened and public satisfaction rose. This period from early 2002 to mid 2005, which coincided with Labour's second term of office, was a time of great success with progress made and acknowledged internally and externally. The NHS was held up as an example to the rest of the public sector of how improvement could be made. The Prime Minister's Delivery Unit and others who had been leaning over our shoulders to mark our homework only the year before now publicised our results.

We had got our act together.

Reform

The initial improvements primarily came through a mixture of tough top-down performance management, imaginative service re-design and extra resources. However, it had become increasingly clear that the top-down management envisaged in the NHS Plan wouldn't work by itself at sufficient scale and with sufficient sustainability. We had developed some very effective methods of implementation but found that we needed more levers than we had to hand. The first area of reform – the re-design of services – even when supported with very effective performance management wasn't enough.

As a result of this experience the Government announced a wider reform programme in April 2002 in response to the Wanless Review.[23] This brought in much more radical change involving the creation of Foundation Trusts, competition, markets and the use of the private sector that weren't in the Plan.

These were mainly very uncomfortable for the NHS and were not applauded in the same way by the great and the good of the healthcare world. They hadn't been part of the hopes and aspirations encapsulated in the Plan. These new reforms simply weren't what most of them had thought that they had signed up to with the NHS Plan. Many of the Government's supporters in the Labour Party and elsewhere also opposed them. They set the NHS in a new direction.

These were reforms of the whole system – changing the organisation and the incentives within it as a means of accelerating improvement. Hospitals were given greater autonomy, competition was introduced for providers, patients were offered choices and the way the money flowed in the system was changed so as to reward success.

These reforms resulted in some re-organisation. At the same time the new staff contracts were brought in – as part of the third area of reform, staff restructuring – in order to improve effectiveness and performance. These were difficult to negotiate and proved very complex, and sometimes contentious, to implement.

Reform in the fourth area – knowledge, technology and science – proceeded much more quietly and with less controversy. A new R and D strategy was developed and NICE expanded its role into wider areas of providing evidence for the NHS and its decision makers.

All these changes were made with the long term intention of embedding improvement and making it self-sustaining rather than dependent on the guiding and, sometimes, heavy hand of management. We attempted to move as smoothly as possible from a 80:20 top down management system to a 20:80 bottom up one over this period.

Figure 3.1 shows the four areas of reform. The next four chapters each describe one of these areas and show how their combination accelerated improvement.

Most of the progress had been made with health services rather than with public health and as this period progressed a new emphasis was given to the very different task of tackling public health issues such as diet, smoking and exercise; strengthening engagement with patients; and making better links with all those organisations dealing with social services and education which affected health and were part of the wider health system.

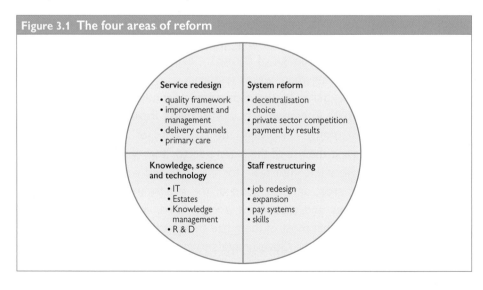

Figure 3.1 The four areas of reform

Service redesign
- quality framework
- improvement and management
- delivery channels
- primary care

System reform
- decentralisation
- choice
- private sector competition
- payment by results

Knowledge, science and technology
- IT
- Estates
- Knowledge management
- R & D

Staff restructuring
- job redesign
- expansion
- pay systems
- skills

Over-stretch, recovery and next stages

The very successful period lasted for more than three years but contained the seeds of its own downfall. Eventually the combination of all these changes led to over-stretch and a loss of momentum. The enthusiasm that had marked the start of the NHS plan had been dissipated. At the same time the NHS was starting to overspend as new capacity came on line, more staff were recruited and organisations geared up for the increased competition they were facing. This was made worse by the fact that with the exception of the Prime Minister all the political members of the leadership group and their advisers changed, and some of the political direction was lost. In this fourth phase from the middle of 2005 to early 2007 improvement stalled and finances got out of control.

In retrospect it is possible to see that a mixture of the complexity of the changes, some loss of overall coherence and the absence of new ideas were too much for the system and its leaders to handle. We lost clear direction and those all important features of political change, the initiative and the momentum to carry us through. At the time, after a rather bungled re-organisation and with finances worsening, I felt that I couldn't command the full support of my NHS colleagues and decided to retire in 2006. It was in some ways a fulfilment of my father's observations six years earlier.

The fifth and final period of these reforms from 2007 to 2010 was one of recovery, consolidation and some re-adjustment of priorities. There was greater emphasis on clinical leadership and quality. My successors – I had been followed, as I had recommended, by two excellent colleagues taking on the roles of Chief Executive and Permanent Secretary separately – brought the finances under control and quietened the situation down. The improvements were maintained and continued but the radical political edge had been lost.

The one big change was heralded by the "Next Stage Review" initiated in June 2007, which the new Prime Minister, Gordon Brown, asked Lord Ara Darzi to lead.[24] Ara brought forward proposals which were designed to strengthen clinical and local ownership and move on more firmly from the top down and more managerial and politically dominated period. Clinical governance had been introduced in 1998 to ensure that organisations concentrated on quality of care; organisations were now expected to prepare quality accounts and pay as much attention to quality as to finance.

By 2009 the NHS had begun to look, just as it had in 1995 and 1996, towards the next Government, whoever that might be and whatever it might bring.

The cumulative effect of all these changes was that the NHS finished the first decade of the 21st century far stronger than it started it. It was improved on almost all measures of performance and was beginning to show good comparisons with other similar nations.

None of us working in the NHS were, of course, satisfied with where we had got to. It was an improvement but there was so much more to do as we will discuss later. Nevertheless, the NHS had turned a corner and the Conservative Party went into the 2010 Election pledging to support and improve the NHS.

Conclusions and key points

1. The creation and launch of the NHS Plan was a very successful exercise in getting Prime Ministerial, cross Government and stakeholder support as well as funding for a major transformation programme.

2. The Plan set a clear direction and was very ambitious with more than 200 targets of different sorts – for inputs, service improvements and health outcomes. The number of targets and an inherent tension between a top down and a bottom up approach were to be problems in the years to come.

3. Mobilisation takes time and there was a significant lag of more than a year before results started to come through. This was both frustrating and problematic. The Government resorted to a series of small scale initiatives to maintain momentum during this period.

4. The NHS had to deal both with the day to day management of services as well as with more unusual events like Public Inquiries at the same time as introducing reforms. Success in managing "winter pressures" helped build confidence whilst waiting for results.

5. At the outset and in order to kick start change, there needed to be very firm leadership and very clear accountability, particularly in an organisation like the NHS which was in practice very decentralised and had many different leaders.

6. Firm leadership and service re-design were not enough by themselves and more radical system reforms were introduced which took the NHS and many of the Government's natural supporters out of their comfort zone and caused a great deal of controversy.

7. The mixture of the four areas of reform – service re-design, system reform, staff restructuring and better use of knowledge, science and technology – complimented each other and accelerated change.

8. The combination of so many changes at once; overspending; changes in leadership; and a poorly conceived reorganisation created a major set of problems after five years. This was followed by a period of recovery. Improvement continued with a new emphasis on clinical leadership and quality but the radical edge had disappeared from policy.

References

1. Department of Health (2000) *The NHS Plan – A plan for investment, A plan for reform*, Cmd 4818-1, The Stationery Office.
2. Ibid. p 10.
3. Ibid. p 17.
4. Ibid. pp 10 and 134.
5. Ibid. p 135.
6. Ibid. p 130.
7. Ibid. p 120.
8. Derek Wanless (2002) *Our future health: taking a long-term view;* HM Treasury, April.
9. Ibid p 35.
10. Ibid.
11. Department of Health (2000) *The NHS Plan – A plan for investment, A plan for reform;* Cmd 4818-1, The Stationery Office, p 132.
12. Edwards B and Fall M (2005) *The Executive Years of the NHS – The England Account 1985–2003*, Radcliffe.
13. Department of Health: NHS Plan Implementation Programme.
14. Kotter JP (1996) *Leading change*. Harvard Business School Press.
15. Department of Health (1998) *A first class service: quality in the NHS;* July.
16. See Chapter 7 for a discussion of the wider role played in later years by NICE.
17. Department of Health (2000) *The NHS Cancer Plan – a plan for investment, a plan for reform;* 27th Sept.
18. Edwards B and Fall M (2005) *The Executive Years of the NHS – The England Account 1985–2003*, Radcliffe.
19. Department of Health (2001) *Shifting the balance of power – securing delivery.*
20. 46th Report of Parliamentary Accounts Committee.
21. Department of Health (2002) *Emergency care report 2001–2002: how the NHS and its partner agencies managed emergency services during winter 2001–2002;* 10 April.
22. Department of Health (2002) *Chief Executive's Report to the NHS April 2001–March 2002;* 10th April.
23. Department of Health (2002) *Delivering the NHS Plan: next steps for investment, next steps for reform;* CM5503, 18 April.
24. Department of Health (2008) *Our NHS, Our future: NHS next stage review – leading local changes*, 9 May.

Chapter 4

Service improvement and delivery

"We didn't believe you were really serious about reducing waiting times until the second year", a senior doctor told me later.

He and his colleagues knew that every new Government sets out to reduce waiting lists when they take up office. It generally lasted a year until "events", normally in the shape of a difficult winter with increased emergency work, blew them off course. We had all seen "waiting list initiatives before" and watched waiting lists fall for a period only to rise, seemingly inevitably, again. He wasn't being particularly cynical; history showed that his was the genuine voice of experience.

We stuck it out and the results started to come through – to the relief of the politicians and me. In my first annual report to the NHS in April 2002 I was at last able to report with confidence that we were on track across almost all of our main target areas. As this quotation about inpatient waiting times shows, however, we still had a long way to go.

> *"At 31 March 2001 10,400 patients had been waiting more than 15 months for admission and about 80,000 patients waited more than 15 months during the year.*
> *At 31 March 2002 preliminary figures show that two patients have been waiting more than 15 months. Both will be admitted as soon as possible. In both cases there have been special circumstances."*[1]

These 2000/2001 figures seem unbelievably awful today. 80,000 people had waited more than 15 months for hospital admission during the previous year! This wait was only after the surgeon had decided to admit them – they might have had to wait for another year before that for an outpatient appointment.

No wonder the public were demanding change.

These figures show how bad the NHS had become. The sad truth was that in 2000 we – clinicians and managers alike – had become used to very poor standards and there was a feeling of inevitability about long surgical waiting lists. For some people they were synonymous with the NHS and they certainly drove an expansion in private medicine.

A deeper look at the 2000/2001 figures showed that urgent cases were generally admitted quickly and that the median waiting time for inpatient admission was 12.9 weeks. There was however a very long tail of patients waiting much longer than this and significant numbers waiting up to the limit then of 78 weeks or 18 months.

The same pattern was true in the time spent waiting for an outpatient appointment with a median time of 4.8 weeks and a maximum of 52 weeks.[2]

This analysis suggests that the NHS was prioritising at least some cases and supports the popular idea that the NHS is at its best in dealing with the urgent and the serious. Indeed whatever the position on waiting lists it wasn't all terrible. It is worth remembering that the best UK hospitals are in the NHS, not the private sector, with wonderful institutions like Great Ormond St, the Royal Marsden, the Freeman, Addenbrookes and the Oxford Radcliffe to name just a few. There was excellent medicine practiced and excellent care given in many hospitals, clinics and surgeries for much of the time. In making improvements the NHS had a great deal to build on as well as a great deal to do. It wasn't a hopeless case.

However, if you had a common complaint – cataracts, a hernia, or varicose veins – you might well find yourself waiting a very long time. These might not be clinically urgent conditions but a life enhancing cataract operation for an 80 year old is urgent in another more human sense.

The NHS Plan set targets for 2005 of maximum inpatient waiting times reducing to six months and outpatient waiting to 13 weeks. Later, in 2004 when good progress was being made these were re-set for a maximum total – combining the outpatient and inpatient elements – of 18 weeks to be achieved in 2010.

All these targets were successfully met and median waiting times fell to 4.3 weeks for inpatients and 2.7 weeks for outpatients, despite the fact that the total numbers of patients treated rose from 17 to 19 million a year over this period.[3]

The numbers of people waiting also fell from a high of 1.3 million in 1998 to 821,000 in 2005 and 633,000 in 2010.[4] It was becoming more like an appointment book with three months of patients scheduled than an out of control waiting list.

The 2005 targets seemed unachievable to many people at the time; whilst the actual achievement of 2010 would have been simply unbelievable. The scale of the challenge is shown in Figure 4.1.

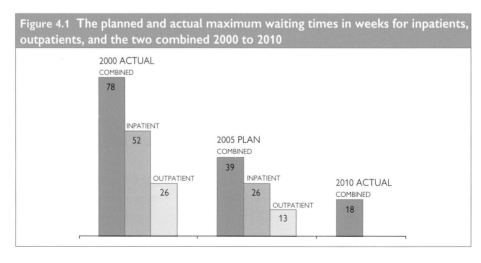

Figure 4.1 The planned and actual maximum waiting times in weeks for inpatients, outpatients, and the two combined 2000 to 2010

Waiting – whether for admission to hospital, to see a GP, for an outpatient appointment, for an ambulance to arrive, to be given "clot busting" drugs after a suspected heart attack, or in A and E – was the highest profile public issue. The NHS Plan responded with targets for improvement in all of them. There were also targets for inputs such as increases in particular types of operations and in staffing. It wasn't all just about process and inputs; there were also stretching targets for reducing premature deaths from cancer and coronary heart diseases and reducing suicide rates.

This chapter looks at how we went about securing delivery through management and quality improvement processes. It discusses the setting and use of targets as well as giving examples of improvements across the spectrum. It also describes the many new ways that people could access help from the NHS. It was no longer just through the old routes of GPs or A and E.

Delivery was greatly supported by having more staff, equipment and money, as described in Chapters 6, 7 and 8; but success also depended very much on how they were used.

Securing delivery

My approach as Chief Executive was to combine a focus on results with an inclusiveness that was intended to enable as many people as possible to lead and make their contribution.

Over time this was mirrored in the way I used the Delivery Directorate and the Modernisation Agency to create a two part delivery process. On the one hand was the tough accountability of performance management and on the other support for creativity and innovation. On the one hand we made it clear what performance improvements were expected, on the other we helped people to achieve them.

The amount of attention that any NHS organisation received from the performance management part depended on how well it was performing. The best performers saw less of the performance managers and had much more freedom of action. The poorer performers received a lot of attention. The support they received from the Modernisation Agency part depended on what they needed. Sometimes, of course, we got this balance wrong; but the general approach was sustained through these years.

As the more centralised and streamlined accountability arrangements in the NHS came into effect these two levers became very powerful and effective. At the outset of the period, however, the structures were just bedding in and we still had to contend with some real psychological and cultural barriers to improvement.

Raising standards and raising expectations

The psychological barriers to progress were real. Some people had got used to poor standards and failings. They were also used to politically led waiting list and other initiatives running out steam. There were demoralising attacks from the media and, as always some people with a vested interest in failure. There were even some well rehearsed intellectual arguments for why things couldn't get better.

One argument, still quite common today, is that long waiting is unavoidable in a service that is free at the point of need and is a legitimate means of managing a fixed budget. This is only partially true. There are many other levers. Faster treatment is one of them. It can reduce complications, stop acute conditions becoming chronic and thereby save costs. In any case the extreme situation in 2000 was not just the result of the ebbs and flows of managing a fixed budget, it revealed that waiting time simply wasn't a priority for the service and wasn't being managed.

On the other hand there were very loud demands for improvement and action coming from patients, the politicians and the media.

We tackled the psychological barriers in three ways, although we didn't describe it or see it quite so clearly as this at the time. Firstly, more money eased the pressure whilst three year budgeting allowed the NHS to plan expenditure better. Secondly, and most controversially, we gave the service some major top-down shocks to get it moving – primarily through a policy of publicly "naming and shaming" the worst performers coupled with a very much tougher approach to holding people to account for performance. Thirdly, examples of what could be done were identified and given a great deal of publicity as we developed mechanisms for re-designing services and spreading good practice.

Star ratings – a shock to the system

We introduced a star rating scheme in 2001 through which the newly formed and independent Commission for Health Improvement (CHI) gave acute trusts zero, one, two or three stars on their cumulative performance on a list of 21 activities in four domains: key targets, clinical focus, patient focus and staff focus.[5] It gave a major shock to the system.

Those that got no stars – there were 12 in the first year– were subject to a great deal of attention, had to implement improvement plans and in some cases had major management changes. Those that achieved three stars were given more freedom from scrutiny – so called "earned autonomy" – and access to a performance fund and other benefits.

The NHS generally hated it. Those who came out at the top – there were 35 three star hospitals out of the nearly 200 assessed in that first year – felt vindicated and enjoyed the praise lavished on them by Ministers and the media; but there was a great deal of criticism of methodology and many accusations of unfairness. Many clinicians were incensed that their hospital was being measured on what they saw as mostly managerial or administrative criteria which ignored the clinical excellence of their particular service.

The methodologies for assessment and the choice of criteria were the best we had to hand at the time and, I believe, were applied fairly and independently. The point was not to achieve a perfect assessment model first time – which would not have been possible – but to start a process of scrutiny, whereby a Trust was judged by external people not self-assessed, and to open up the debate with the public. It raised all kinds of uncomfortable questions: why were two hospitals that appeared very similar performing very differently; how could you claim to have an excellent clinical service in a hospital that was dirty, had long waiting lists and failed to manage its budget; how could senior clinicians think they had no responsibility for this; and why were some Chief Executives paid so highly for apparent failure?

These questions needed to be asked and the problems they identified needed to be dealt with.

Over time CHI and its successors improved their methodologies and widened the system to include other types of organisations including Ambulance, Community and Mental Health Trusts and Primary Care Trusts. They eventually moved away from the star rating system in 2005 and introduced a more rounded and sophisticated report card, rather as had been envisaged in the original Plan.[6]

Star rating was not the only method of "naming and shaming" and from time to time lists were – and still are – published of the best and worst Trusts in terms of death rates or cleanliness. It is only the lists of the worst performers, of course, that attract any real attention in the media. Some people and some organisations were treated very savagely indeed in the media with all manner of hurtful accusations thrown at them from being incompetent to being uncaring or venal.

Star rating was crude, could in some ways be unfair and left a number of bruised people in its wake but I would defend it as the right approach for the particular time. It gave an appropriate shock to the system which made people take notice and take action about long standing problems. None of what was revealed was new. However, its exposure to the wider gaze of the public and the rough handling of the media undoubtedly was a new development. It was one of many instances during this period – others were the Bristol, Alder Hey and Shipman Inquiries – when things that had previously been hidden were brought into the light and helped shift the culture of the NHS.

The separation of Trusts into different bands of performance was, of course, also very true to life. Some did do better than others and in looking at good practice we could see that some were ahead of the field. These were the early adopters who often designed the best practice. The majority followed them; whilst another small minority made up the laggards and the real problem cases.

Quality improvement and the re-design of services

The Modernisation Agency (MA), which had been created in 2001 to identify and spread good practice, developed programmes to support Trusts operating at these different performance levels. The zero star Trusts and others identified as having major problems received a great deal of remedial attention; whilst high performers were watched and supported as they led the way in developing good practice.

Star rating was part of the tough accountability side of our management style whilst the MA was at the centre of the supportive, helpful part. The MA assisted in developing models for re-designing services, demonstrated what success looked like and in doing so helped build confidence that improvement was possible.

There were other supportive aspects too and there were incentives for innovation. High performing organisations were first in line for new investment: we wanted to reward success not failure. They were also praised publicly, invited to Prime Ministerial receptions and some of their leaders were given state honours. It is sometimes overlooked how effective public recognition is as a motivator. Tony Blair regularly offered his support, coming to occasional management meetings to help maintain momentum.

Even the most senior and the most cynical can be touched by the magic and the power of high office. I have lost track of the number of times I have heard "… *and as the Prime Minister said* …", *"What people were saying in Downing St last week* …" and sometimes *"As Tony said to me"*…. I have no doubt that the people exposed to this sort of attention went home after such a meeting and told their family and friends about it. I certainly did.

The MA was an exciting place to work. It was at the forefront of innovation, was full of interesting people and a place to share ideas and be inspired by others. It ran programmes on improving services and collaboratives for sharing best practice on many topics from orthopaedics to hearts and eyes and, through the Leadership Centre, offered training and development for individuals and groups. The MA was always very open and welcoming and anyone could become part of it by becoming an MA Associate once they had been on a programme. In doing so they joined a movement for improvement, were kept up to date and had the chance to communicate and meet with others in order to share and learn.

It made a practice of learning from elsewhere as well as from the NHS: whether it was *6 Sigma*, *Lean thinking* or other approaches to service re-design and improvement. In particular, the MA and its successors gained, and still gain, a great deal from the Institute for Healthcare Improvement (IHI) – its then President, Don Berwick, was part of the Modernisation Board in 2000 – and Maureen Bisognano, now the President, and colleagues still play a supporting role in all four UK countries.

An example shows how the MA worked at its best. There were, as I described in Chapter 2, major problems in A and E Departments in the late 90s. They were acting as a pressure valve for the whole system: as long as patients were kept in trolleys in A and E it meant that the hospital wards and the GPs could operate reasonably normally. Improvement was desperately needed.

There were four linked interventions. Firstly, a target was set of ensuring that by December 2004 all A and E patients were seen, treated, admitted or discharged within four hours of arrival. Later we reduced this to 98%, recognising that there would be some exceptions for clinical reasons. Importantly, this was a target for the whole Trust and the whole NHS system so everyone had some responsibility for ensuring that patient flows into and through the hospital were improved. It was no longer just a problem for the Department. The local NHS collectively was expected to produce plans and trajectories showing how they would achieve the target. They would be performance managed on this by the Delivery Directorate.

Secondly, money was made available to make physical improvements in each Department. Thirdly, the MA was given the responsibility of creating and implementing an appropriate methodology for improvement. Finally, a National Clinical director or Czar was appointed.

Sir George Alberti, the just retired President of the Royal College of Physicians, provided clinical leadership for the implementation of the *Emergency Services Collaborative* in September 2002. He set about the role – which he described as that of *"trolley Czar"* – with great vigour. Although the A and E target was achieved on time at the end of 2004, George remained in post until 2009 constantly seeking ways to help make further improvements in the quality of care that A and E attenders and other emergency and urgent patients received.

In preparation for the launch of the collaborative the MA had gone through a process of identifying best practice in A and E departments around the country. One of the best ideas they discovered from hospitals around the country was "*See and Treat*". Traditionally patients in an A and E Department would be seen first by the most junior staff and be passed on from a clerical person to a nurse to a junior doctor and, possibly, eventually reach a Consultant. *See and Treat* turned this upside down. The first person who saw them was the most senior on duty at the time. Because of their experience they were able to make much quicker decisions and order fewer tests and so on. It worked very effectively.

The MA took this and other observations about what was most effective and set up a programme using the methodology of the *Breakthrough Collaborative* developed by IHI. This has many parts but at its heart are three concepts: the *PDSA* cycle of improvement, an understanding of the importance of data and measurement and the notion that parallel learning between organisations can accelerate change.

The *PDSA* cycle – plan, do study, act – is based on the idea that in trying to make a large scale improvement it is best to start with a single element rather than trying to design the whole change in detail from the start.[7] So in trying to improve their Department a team would be asked to identify one change that might help, put it into practice for a period, see what happened and amend, abandon or keep it as appropriate – in other words plan, do, study and act. They would then do another change and so on. Crucially, they would measure impact in an objective way using data they could track: subjective perceptions were not enough.

A *Collaborative* involves several units trying to make improvements in the same area at the same time and learning from each others successes and failures. Thus five A and E teams might each be working on improving their Departments. One might conclude that a change in staff rostering would help and try it. Another might trial nurses ordering X rays; another faster access to social services or to pathology test results and so on. Working in parallel they could learn from each other and from the pre-work done by the MA on *See and Treat* and other practices.

The MA used this methodology in cancer, coronary heart disease and other areas. In A and E there were six successive waves of Departments working collaboratively, starting with 30 Trusts in October 2002. Figure 4.2 shows how successful they were. There are many very significant points about this approach including the fact that change came bottom up from the actual participants themselves. This was very important. I cannot imagine that if the NHS Chief Executive, or even the Chief Medical Officer, had told Consultants and senior nurses that they must be the first people to see patients in their Department that this would have happened consistently and at scale. However, because they decided to do so for themselves, all Departments adopted a variant of this methodology with senior doctors and nurses taking their turn as the first people to greet patients at the front door.

I described earlier how powerless I felt as Chief Executive of the Oxford Radcliffe as I tried to improve my A and E. Later on as Regional Director I came back from my Friday visits in South East England and London horrified by conditions in some of our A and E Departments. This programme and continuing attention from George Alberti and others improved them almost beyond recognition.

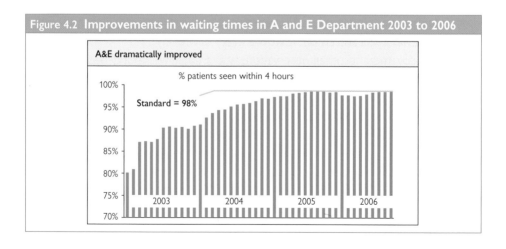

Figure 4.2 **Improvements in waiting times in A and E Department 2003 to 2006**

Most A and E Departments now have good systems and processes. They are still, six years after it was first achieved, meeting the four hour target – even though 1½ million more people a year now use this improved service.

The Emergency Services Collaborative was just one of many successful improvement projects carried out by the MA. It also published and spread ideas about improvement. One of the most important publications was "*10 High Impact changes for service improvement and delivery*" which brought together some of its most important learning about how to improve quality and costs.[8] We built this into the formal NHS planning process and expected all organisations to review the list and apply the findings as appropriate. Over time, however, the MA became really too successful for its own good as an institution. It grew fast and attracted many of the brightest and most self-motivated people and in so doing started to drain the talent from the front line. I received complaints from Chief Executives of Trusts and PCTs that they were losing their best people to work on innovation in the MA when they really needed them to do the hard day to day work of delivery in their hospitals and units. They wanted the MA to identify best practice, train, develop and inspire their people but not to take them away from the front line.

We were beginning to move towards decentralisation and therefore changed our approach. We gave greater emphasis to building improvement capacity locally within the operational units, pared down the central MA and in 2005 replaced it with the much smaller NHS Institute for Improvement and Innovation (the NHS Institute). The action for improvement had moved to where it was most needed in support of the front line whilst the Institute maintained a more strategic national role in identifying innovation and drawing in ideas from abroad.

The MA was not the only vehicle which helped "modernise" the NHS: management institutes, universities and training centres around the countries fed in ideas; a GP, Sir John Oldham, as we will see later, set up the National Primary Care Development Team (NPDT) to bring improvements in primary care. We even had an abortive attempt to create an NHS University. This was a time of experimentation and a search for what worked.

These improvement programmes have left a great deal behind them and are reflected today not just in the continuing work of the NHS Institute but also in the current QIPP – Quality, Innovation, Productivity, Prevention – programme designed to support clinical teams and which is staffed by some of the leaders from the earlier wave of improvement including John Oldham and Helen Bevan. Over the last 10 years a real quality movement has developed in England.

I invited David Fillingham, the MA Chief Executive in that heady period from 2002 to 2005, to look back from the vantage point of 2011. He said that:

> *"The biggest legacy of the Modernisation Agency is the hundreds of people who worked in it and the thousands who worked with it who learned new skills and are still using them today. It was very successful in bringing clinicians and managers together locally to make change."*

Whatever the particular structures adopted, my experience with the MA and the other groups and programmes was that it is essential to have some from of systematic process of quality improvement in any health system and to ensure that it is well integrated into the management process.

The two handed approach

The excitement and innovation of quality improvement was matched by the daily grind of getting results. It is difficult to overemphasise the amount of persistence and attention to detail that is required to pursue a goal doggedly over time and the discipline this requires.

John Bacon who was responsible for the Delivery Directorate and his colleagues encapsulated this approach in the four box diagram shown in Figure 4.3. It starts in box 1 with clear goals, measurement and accountability; goes on in box 2 to identify the evidence and best practice and secure buy in; moves on in box 3 to ensure there is performance management and that learning from the early stages of delivery is fed back into later stages; and continues in box 4 by providing support for high risk organisations. It combined quality improvement and accountability.

It worked.

Targets

The Labour Government brought a new discipline to public services with an insistence on target setting, measurement and delivery. Whatever the particular language and approach, something of this kind was clearly needed or we would continue to see public services drift and decline.

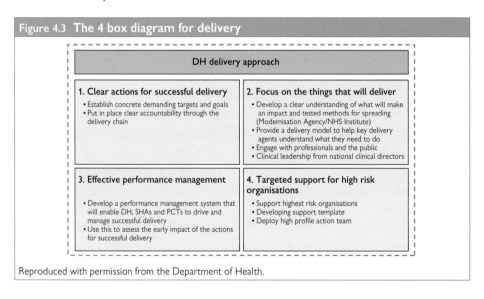

Figure 4.3 The 4 box diagram for delivery

Reproduced with permission from the Department of Health.

All forms of priority setting have their downsides and their detractors. There will be things which aren't prioritised: some attention needs to be paid to the non-priorities so they don't get worse whilst concentration is elsewhere. Some people will focus too narrowly on the target and miss the point. A lot of GPs appear to have treated their target – that everyone should be able to get an appointment with a clinician in their practice within 48 hours – as meaning that no appointments could be booked after that date for follow ups and so on. Others, too, seems to have missed the fact that the real aim of the NHS Plan was to eliminate unnecessary waiting and make traditional surgical waiting lists *"a thing of the past"*.[9]

Priority setting can also make people game play, hitting the goal by manoeuvring, not making real change; and it can make them cheat as I knew all too painfully from my appearance at the PAC in January 2002 (see Chapter 3).

We could have done better at managing all these things but the upside of targets was also enormous. In the pre-target NHS that I took over in 2000 about 4% of heart patients died whilst on the waiting list for surgery. We therefore targeted heart waiting lists for faster reductions than other specialities and reduced mortality on the waiting list to zero – more than 5,500 waited more than three months for heart surgery in 2000, but no one did in 2005.

In 2000 only 24% of patients received "clot busting" drugs within an hour of a heart attack despite the evidence of their effectiveness being available for almost 20 years. The use of targets together with management action and service re-design increased that to 55% by March 2005.[10] Delivery of these two cardiac targets helped save many lives.

England, alone of the four UK countries, set targets from the outset. External researchers have shown that, with the same boost in funding for all four countries, the English NHS improved fastest. Some didn't improve at all until targets and similar methodologies were introduced.[11]

There has been a lot of debate and controversy about targets. The problem in the NHS was that the NHS Plan overdid it. There were too many targets, some were badly conceived and designed and we weren't always good enough at changing direction when we needed to and in managing their downside and their, mostly malign, unintended consequences. External opinion now, however, seems to be moving towards saying that targets were useful – as one management tool amongst others – but that *"systems need to be put in place to minimise gaming to meet targets and ensure targets are not causing unwanted effects elsewhere"*.[12] It seems to me to be the right judgement.

The current Government has, however, listened to the critics and taken the populist decision to abolish targets. Standards are already slipping in waiting times and elsewhere. I imagine that they will find some way to replace them before we slip back to anywhere near the dreadful position of the 1990's.

How NHS services changed

Targets aren't the whole story. Activity levels grew, the range of services offered expanded and quality improved.

Figures for the end of March 2005 show that over the five year period since March 2000 – just before the launch of the NHS Plan – there were large increases in all the traditional types of NHS activity. Elective hospital admissions went up by ½ million (11%); attendances at the major Accident and Emergency facilities increased by 1½ million (12%); emergency ambulance journeys went up by ½ million (almost 20%); and the number of first outpatient attendances at hospitals increased by more than 1.3 million (11%).[13]

This expansion was partly due to growth in capacity with more NHS staff and more facilities; but a part was also due to the reduction in waiting times drawing in more people. A further part was there were now a much wider range of channels through which members of the public could access help. This was one of the most significant changes during this period.

New services were created such as NHS Direct (a nurse led telephone advice service) which was being used by 6½ million people annually by 2005; NHS Direct Online had more than 9 million hits by that time; Walk in Centres dealing with minor injuries were being used by 2 million people; Treatment Centres which dealt with a limited number of high volume procedures were just being introduced, some of them run by private companies; and the numbers of procedures undertaken outside hospital, the number of outreach service interventions and prescriptions written in the community all increased as result of specific policies.[14] In addition GPs were increasingly able to send their patients directly to "*Open Access*" services such as radiology, endoscopy and physiotherapy without first being seen by a hospital doctor.

Another part of the increase was due to new services reaching more people. NHS Direct Online for example was used by more young men – an easily missed target of much health promotion work – and Walk In Centres at railway stations and in town centres were more convenient for many people, particularly those commuters who worked at any distance from their home and their GP.

There were complaints from some clinicians that none of the interventions reduced pressure on their hospitals but only raised public expectations. It was an important point: not least because people did begin to expect more of the NHS. This, of course, was a good thing: standards had become far too low in far too many areas. Nevertheless, we did want to see pressure and activity move away from hospitals. The figures show that this was happening to an extent: the biggest increases in elective surgery undertaken in hospital were in the first few of these years – as we reduced waiting lists – and by 2005 they had levelled off.

The various policies that had put GPs and Primary Care into the pivotal planning and funding role in the NHS, from Fund Holding in the 1990s to PCTs and beyond, have all tried to tackle this issue. Typically they are involved in re-shaping and not just reducing hospital activity. A PCT or GP Practice might well want to see some increases in referrals to hospital for particular specialities, such as cardiology and oncology, but reductions in others such as orthopaedics where patients can be well managed in their local care. The overall effect may be little change in numbers but a big change in effectiveness.

This period saw a flowering in the type and range of NHS services in an attempt to reach everybody and, though this was mostly implicit rather than explicit, to offer more services that the public liked and thereby increase support for the NHS. This is an important point that is not just about party politics.

A public service like the NHS needs to market itself and make sure its customers are satisfied. Failure and ruin may come quicker in a private sector setting but during this period the future of the NHS was very uncertain and the prospect of failure was real. It needed friends and it needed to be seen to be improving. NHS Direct, Walk In Centres and Treatment Centres were all very visible and more popular with the public than the professions.

Figure 4.4 gives an outline of the range of services on offer and describes the results we achieved.

Figure 4.4 The changing NHS – faster more convenient services[15]

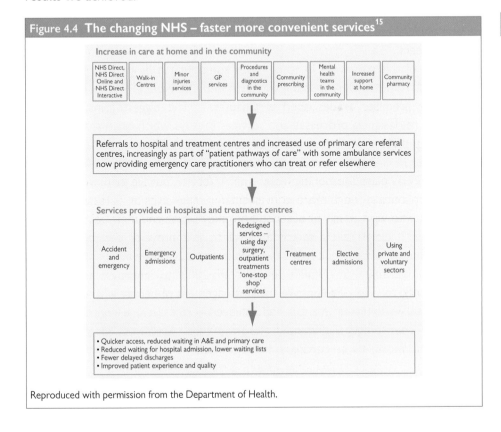

Reproduced with permission from the Department of Health.

Primary care

Primary care has increasingly taken on a bigger role in recent years both as service provider and as planner and commissioner. It is the front door and perhaps "shop window" for the NHS as a whole. There are around 300 million consultations a year in GPs surgeries, meaning that on average every member of the population goes to their family doctor about six times a year.

There were very big problems at the start of this period with gaining fast access to GPs, particularly in inner city areas, and so the NHS Plan included "*must do*" targets of "*guaranteed access to a primary care professional within 24 hours and to a primary care doctor within 48 hours by 2004*".[16]

Sir John Oldham, himself a GP, took control of these targets. He set up a network of 11 regionally based GP leaders and started to work with GPs to improve performance. The presenting problem was that in most practices there appeared to be too many patients wanting too many appointments for the slots available. It looked like a simple problem of resources and that, indeed, was how most GPs saw it.

Closer examination, however, showed that in many cases there were problems of scheduling: staffing levels were the same for every session throughout the week and weren't related to demand, even though patients came in easily identified peaks; special clinics were booked on Mondays, the busiest day, when more general clinics were needed; and doctors were doing routine tasks which could be done by others.

Problems of this sort were in some cases compounded by poor premises and lack of staff. Some extra resourcing was provided and NHS LIFT was established to improve premises as described in Chapter 7. The biggest gains, however, came from re-designing processes and services in ways which once again owed a lot to IHI and were similar to those used by the MA. There were differences, however.

Many clinicians played leadership roles in MA activity, but Sir John and his team worked very much through clinician to clinician relationships at as local a level as possible. It was very much about primary care improvement by primary care professionals. It didn't have a specific brief to build improvement capacity as the MA did; although, of course, it had a big impact in this area as well.

John and his team at NDPT set out in 2000 to improve access and, simultaneously, to help GPs improve their management of people with established heart disease. Within four years it had achieved a 76% average improvement in access and contributed significantly, alongside other initiatives, to a four fold reduction in mortality in coronary heart disease. They moved on to tackle diabetes and chronic lung diseases as well as running an award-winning programme where residents of deprived areas were themselves the improvement teams – the Healthy Communities Collaborative – which reduced falls in older people by 32%.

Ten years on Sir John Oldham says *"we started with angry GPs standing up in meetings pointing fingers at me saying I was just a government lackey, and ended 44 months later with having engaged 5500 practices and transformed services for 32 million people"*.

The results were impressive and the access targets were met. The measure that was used for waiting times to see a GP was the waiting time for the *"third available appointment"*. This eliminated special circumstances which might exist for the first available one such as a cancellation by a patient. Figure 4.5 shows how waiting times dropped for four successive waves of practices. It also shows that the later waves improved more quickly that the earlier ones. This was a phenomenon we observed with other improvements.

The system itself was learning. This isn't as mysterious or metaphysical as it may sound. People talked to each other in the NHS. GPs or A and E Consultants told each other what they were doing. The networks – which are so strong in health – networked in their normal way to spread news, gossip and learning around the NHS. In pure research terms our controls were contaminated as results leaked out and influenced the behaviour of others not in the original wave. In management terms it was wonderful news.

This system learning is a very important phenomenon. It can be positive or negative and can spread bad news, bad gossip and bad practice just as it can spread the good. It points to the fact that implementers of any change need to take account of and try to influence the social networks and informal organisational structures as well as the formal lines and connections on the organisational chart.

MRSA

The NHS Plan set many targets but missed one vital one. Looking back at the NHS Plan consultation it is clear that the public were concerned about infection control as well as clean hospitals. For whatever reason, it was missed off the list of top priorities and came back to haunt us. It was a real problem and not just a perceived one. Infection control practices had been neglected and infection rates were too high.

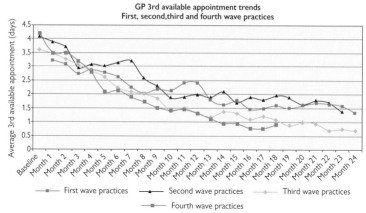

Figure 4.5   Improvements in primary care: showing how the waiting time for the third available appointment improved faster for successive waves

Infection control, and particularly MRSA, was the single issue that did the most damage to the reputation of the NHS during this entire period. John Reid came into office in 2003 having been told in the lobbies of the Commons by fellow MPs that this was the biggest concern they heard from their constituents. The focus at last began to shift and when Dame Christine Beasley was appointed as Chief Nursing Officer (CNO) the following year she found that it was top of her agenda.

Once again we followed the now familiar processes of setting a measurable target, putting in place monitoring and improvement processes, developing expertise and persistently and doggedly pursuing improvement. Once again there was a slow start whilst systems bedded in and we waited anxiously for progress. Once again there was controversy over the target which we had set as a 50% reduction in blood borne MRSA infections despite the only available evidence suggesting that only 15% was achievable. Once again the NHS overachieved with a fall of 75% by 2011.

The CNO and colleagues later took the same approach with *Clostridium difficile* and had similar success. There is some evidence that taking on MRSA in this way helped improve hospital cleanliness, reduced the spread of other infections and improved the standard of patient care at the same time. One target helped hit many goals. The improvement is now embedded in local practice and sustained in the NHS without national support.

Reductions in premature mortality

Our targets to reduce premature deaths before the age of 75 from coronary heart disease by 40% by 2010 and from cancer by 20% compared to a base line of 1995 were tackled in the same way with collaboratives, Czars and some extra funding. In both cases, of course, there were complications because action was needed across the whole system from preventative measures and early diagnosis to treatment in primary, secondary and tertiary care, and on to rehabilitation.

Deaths were already falling because of earlier action, particularly in reducing smoking and pollution. However improvements were better than trend and, whilst the 2010 figures are not yet available, it is very likely both targets have been met.

There continues to be a need for big improvements in both these areas where the UK is a relatively poor performer by international standards. However, it is moving up the international league tables.

Action on reducing deaths from suicide by 20%, led by Professor Louis Appleby as the Czar, was approached in the same way and brought social services as well as health into the action. Here the task was even harder because there was an established upward trend which had to be halted and reversed. It was.

It is very difficult to be definitive about cause and effect. An improving economy undoubtedly helped during this period and the rate fell in some other countries but not, for example, in Northern Ireland where there was no suicide prevention strategy. Most significantly it fell in areas we targeted: there was a sharp downturn in the rate in people under 35 and amongst mental health inpatients and prisoners. There is evidence that here too action by hundreds of people throughout the NHS and social care made a very big difference.

External validation of improvement

External validation of improvement came from a surprising source. The use of the private sector for elective inpatient surgery – in other words for the types of surgery covered by the NHS waiting list – had been growing in recent years. This trend peaked in 2002, having risen more sharply between 1998 and 2002, and has subsequently fallen and seems likely to stagnate or fall further.[17] Private sector activity would have fallen even more sharply if it were not for a rise in cosmetic surgery of the sort that the NHS doesn't do.

The public was voting with its feet. I well remember the jubilation with which we greeted the first publication of these figures in 2004 in the Department. We had been told for the last few years by our many critics that the NHS couldn't be improved. Despite all this pessimism, here we were taking patients back from the private sector. It was a sweet moment, a turning point in the battle.

It was also a shock to the private sector which, as I know from discussion with people who were Board members of private health companies at the time, had been making plans for further growth on the easy assumption of NHS failure.

There was an interesting coda to this. In 2004 we sought tenders for private health companies to provide some challenge to incumbent NHS providers. The big UK companies mostly didn't bid or bid very high, not willing to drop their prices to ours. None of them won contracts but instead we turned to overseas providers.

It was another shock to the private sector as we brought competition for them into the UK market. At the next round of contracting the UK companies bid at reasonable levels and won some of the work. They were learning to adapt to the NHS as a significantly improved provider. It was a start of a new relationship.

System reform

This chapter has concentrated on how service re-design, quality improvement and management helped deliver progress. By themselves these processes were effective but limited. We also needed to introduce some system reforms to accelerate change.

Figure 4.6 illustrates this well. It shows that the number of people waiting more than six months for admission fell quarter by quarter to zero by December 2005. There were two significant falls. The first was when patients who had waited more than six months were permitted a choice as to whether to transfer to another hospital for immediate treatment. The second was when the first independent sector treatment centre (ISTC) opened. The NHS responded to both by accelerating improvement.

The next chapter addresses system reform.

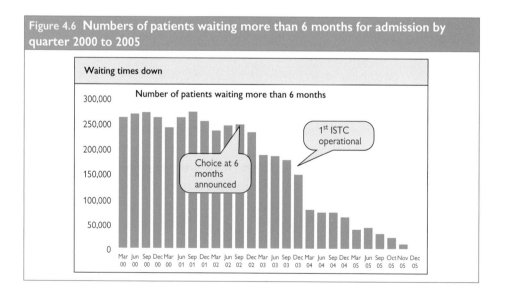

Figure 4.6 Numbers of patients waiting more than 6 months for admission by quarter 2000 to 2005

Conclusions and key points

1. There were enormous improvements in targeted areas. Maximum hospital waiting times fell by three quarters and the median by two thirds. Premature deaths from cancer, coronary heart disease and from suicide fell as planned. New services and new ways of accessing services became available to the public. Activity levels rose very fast as services expanded and improved.

2. Initially there were psychological and confidence barriers to overcome as well as inertia and some opposition. "Star ratings" gave an early shock to the system and helped start improvement.

3. A two part approach of firm performance management and accountability on the one hand and assistance with quality improvement on the other brought results. The innovation of quality improvement needed to be matched with the persistent and daily grind of delivery.

4. A simple model of improvement was developed which involved a clear target and measurement, clinical leadership, knowledge of best practice, local adaptation and clear accountability. It was applied to everything from reducing MRSA to preventing suicides and speeding up services.

5. At its best "the system learned" as the formal mechanisms of communication were aided by informal structures and networks in making improvement. We all learned together.

6. It was important to provide many ways for the public to access services both to improve health but also to secure public support and confidence.

7. As services improved more people used them and the use of the private sector declined – providing external validation of improvement.

8. Improvement could be accelerated by bringing in system reforms alongside the improvement and management processes.

References

1. Department of Health (2002) *Chief Executive's Report to the NHS – April 2001 to March 2002*, April, p 3.
2. Department of Health waiting list statistics – quoted in National Audit Office (2010) Management of NHS Hospital Productivity, 17 Dec .
3. Ibid.
4. Department of Health: *Inpatient and outpatient waiting times/list.*

5. Department of Health (2001) *NHS Performance Ratings: Acute Trusts 2000/01*; Sept.
6. Department of Health (2000) *The NHS Plan – a plan for investment, a plan for reform*; Cmd 4818-1, The Stationary Office.
7. Langley GJ, Moen RD. Nolan KM, Nolan TW, Norman CL, Provost LP (2009) *The Improvement Guide* 2nd edn, Jossey-Bass.
8. NHS Modernisation Agency (2004) *10 High Impact Changes for service improvement and delivery*, Sept.
9. Department of Health (2000) *The NHS Plan – a plan for investment, a plan for reform*; Cmd 4818-1, The Stationary Office, p 19.
10. Ibid. p 41.
11. Bevan G, Hood C (2006) Have targets improved performance in the English NHS? *BMJ*, **332**(7538): 419–22.
12. Ibid.
13. Department of Health (2005) *Chief Executive's Report 2005*; 13 May.
14. Ibid.
15. Ibid. p 13.
16. Department of Health (2000) *The NHS Plan – a plan for investment, a plan for reform*; Cmd 4818-1, The Stationary Office, p 131.
17. Farrington-Douglas J, Coelho MC (2008) *Private Spending on Healthcare*. Institute for Public Policy Research, p 37ff.

Chapter 5

System reforms

It was an error of inexperience.

I was at one of my first major conferences as NHS Chief Executive in the summer of 2001 when I was trapped by a journalist into saying that I saw no reason why the private sector shouldn't provide more services to the NHS. We were in a small screened off area near the main halls: one of those anonymous white spaces which you can find in any conference centre with a few empty tables and chairs littered around waiting for occupants. I was accompanied by a civil servant from the Department's press office who took notes of our conversation.

I was still getting used to the fact that all my public utterances were recorded; having only just discovered that every time I spoke on the phone in my office there was someone in my outer office listening and writing down the key points. When I eventually learned about this I had wondered what I had said in the few weeks when I was unaware of this practice.

It was routine throughout Whitehall, all Ministers and Permanent Secretaries had their calls monitored in this way, and the civil servants had just assumed I knew. It was for my own protection I was told. Nobody would ever be able to claim that I had said something I hadn't. On this occasion the journalist had led me on through gentle questioning. He and the civil servant both wrote my answer down: "*No.*" I agreed. *"I saw no reason why private sector organisations shouldn't tender for this contract."*

Alan Milburn, the Secretary of State, moved fast to repudiate my remarks. A small article appeared in the Financial Times the following day saying that he had criticised me for not following Government policy. The story became one about the Secretary of State overruling the Chief Executive – and not about the use of the private sector at all. He had successfully neutralised the issue.

Milburn was very nervous at the time of even appearing to be doing anything that was outside the Labour orthodoxy on the NHS. He rang me later that day to tell me what he had done. He explained that he had had to fight hard to get agreement across Government for the NHS Plan and its funding and he didn't want anything to jeopardise it. There was already enough political blood on the floor. He didn't say it explicitly, but I suspect his real concern was with the Chancellor and the Treasury who had very fixed views on what the NHS money could be spent on. He wasn't yet ready to alienate them. That would come soon enough.

The use of the private sector had always been a vexed issue for the NHS, whichever party was in power. Like others, when I had been a Trust Chief Executive I had wanted to use a local private hospital as an overflow to help manage the peaks and troughs of my own hospital's work flow. The then Conservative Government didn't like this because of the potential "privatising" message it might send. Whatever they may have believed in private they didn't want the public to have any evidence that they were supporting the private sector rather than the NHS.

Later, as a Regional Director, I had wanted to offer treatment in France to some patients from Kent – which was after all as near as London to the citizens of Dover and Ashford – but had been prevented from doing so. It, too, would not have looked good. The headlines about the NHS not being able to cope would have been very damaging. I imagine the French would have enjoyed it. I know that we were jubilant a few years later when we heard that striking French doctors had hired Wembley Conference Centre for their protest meeting. It was a brilliant negotiating tactic. Unfortunately for us the French Government capitulated. They didn't want their dirty washing exposed in front of les rosbifs. It would no doubt have been a national scandal. Pity! We were looking forward to **those** headlines...

It all seemed, and indeed was, very contradictory when we already used private organisations to do many of the rarer pathology tests and to accommodate and treat a significant number of psychiatric patients. There seemed no practical reason not to expand this use if we could get a better deal for our patients by doing so. Indeed, the NHS Plan itself had proposed a new public/private Concordat to enable the private sector to support NHS modernisation better.[1] There was, however, a pressing political reason.

The Labour Party of which Alan Milburn was a member was still very wedded to an old mental model in which the NHS was seen as a nationalised industry, centrally planned and controlled, and which used only NHS money, staff and facilities to treat NHS patients. There needed to be – and there needed to be seen to be – a cordon sanitaire between the NHS and the private sector. It was a model that was already well out of date by this time because the NHS had already moved on in so many ways. Milburn himself would shortly be the person who would kill it off for good and replace it with a much more modern version of a national health system which, whilst maintaining its founding values and integrity, used the private sector not only as a supplier but also to promote competition and innovation in the NHS.

Time and politics moved on. Within the year we had begun to send a few patients abroad as well as using local private facilities to help reduce waiting lists. Both were explained to the public and the press as temporary measures which showed how seriously we were taking the problem of lack of capacity in the NHS. We were on the front foot, taking the initiative and determined to do what needed doing to improve the service. Alan Milburn was ready to take on old Labour and old attitudes. He had the grace to joke with me in private that he was adopting my policy.

System reform and redesign

I have returned to politics at the start of this chapter because system reform takes us into the political sphere. This chapter is all about the radical system reforms – the system redesign – involved in moving from a nationalised industry to a national health system. This required political will.

There had been great enthusiasm at the launch of the NHS Plan, as we have seen, and a lot of support for redesigning services. In practice many people didn't like the targets and the enhanced accountability that accompanied this. These subsequent system reforms were even further outside the NHS comfort zone. A large part of the Labour Party hated them.

Some of these changes were more successful than others. Together they were the most distinctive feature of this whole period and represented a profound shift for the whole NHS. Starting with decentralisation in 2001 we successively offered patients choice, tendered for the private sector to provide services and introduced new financial incentives.

Over the following years a coherent picture emerged, described successively in policy documents in 2002, 2004 and 2006.[2,3,4] As these three documents show, reform of the NHS had by this time become part of a wider Government approach to reforming public services. This had been initiated shortly after the 2001 election and the public narrative had changed to one where market forces drove improvement.

There were four sets of reforms which, heavily influenced by economists, were described in economic terms as:

- Reforms to the demand side: new commissioning arrangements and the emphasis on promotion of health and prevention of disease would shape demand better; whilst the introduction of patient choice over which services or hospitals they used would make services more personalised and responsive
- Reforms to the supply side: internal competition was promoted as NHS Foundation Trusts were created with greater freedoms; and external competition with non-NHS providers able to enter a more open market
- Transactional reforms: payment by results (PBR) was introduced so that hospitals which attracted the most patients received the most income
- System reforms: new regulation arrangements and changes in staff terms and conditions and in the service contracts with GPs were established to provide the right environment for competition and improvement.

All of these reforms depended on decentralisation of some responsibilities and authority from the Department to more local parts of the NHS and to independent regulators. The next section of this chapter deals with this decentralisation and is followed by sections on each of the four areas of reform in turn.

Figure 5.1 provides a simple visual description of these reforms.

Figure 5.1 The 4 sets of system reforms

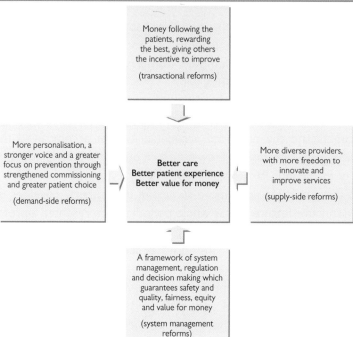

Money following the patients, rewarding the best, giving others the incentive to improve

(transactional reforms)

More personalisation, a stronger voice and a greater focus on prevention through strengthened commissioning and greater patient choice

(demand-side reforms)

**Better care
Better patient experience
Better value for money**

More diverse providers, with more freedom to innovate and improve services

(supply-side reforms)

A framework of system management, regulation and decision making which guarantees safety and quality, fairness, equity and value for money

(system management reforms)

The UK Government's Model of Public Service Reform – A Self-Improving System

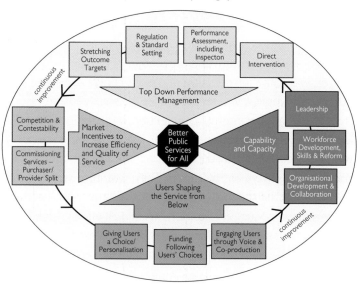

Reproduced with permission from the Department of Health.

Decentralisation – and centralisation

Throughout its history the NHS had had an integrated planning and accountability structure based on geographical units. Health Authorities – at different times these were Area, District or Regional Health Authorities or some mixture of them – were responsible for almost all services in their areas, with the exception of a very few national services. They supervised the activities of the hospitals and other mental health, learning difficulty, community and ambulance units as well as the contracts with GPs, dentists and optometrists. The Health Authorities in turn reported to the Department of Health and ministers. At different times Local Government had been responsible for community services and parts of mental health and public health services; at other times these have been more fully integrated into the NHS (see Appendix 2).

It wasn't quite the top down monolithic organisational structure that its critics have sometimes alleged. The various levels of Health Authorities had their own statutory powers and Local Authorities were accountable to their local electors and not to the national Government. There were often tensions between the different authorities and with the Government. The result was that national plans conceived in Whitehall might take years to be implemented in the cities and counties of the country. Sometimes these tensions were party political with a Health Authority dominated by one political party challenging the policies and decisions of a national Government of a different political colour. Sometimes they would be about local issues and sometimes purely personality driven.

National government did, however, have powerful tools to control the NHS. It allocated the money. It had technical knowledge, issuing circulars about how services needed to be organised. It controlled the national pay negotiations with the unions which set wages and salaries for all health workers. It had patronage with the right to appoint Chairmen and members to the Health Authorities.

It also had the moral authority, and with it the burden, of the expectations of the public and voters. This was a **National** Health Service and the Secretary of State of the day was seen as the person responsible.

These arrangements weren't efficient. They were a compromise which attempted not only to balance off all the competing interests at the different levels; but to recognise the protected position of some of the unions and the leadership role of the doctors, nurses and administrators. It was a recipe for inaction with different groups having in effect a right of veto over change. It is not surprising that successive Governments re-organised the NHS trying to find the optimum arrangement.[5]

Labour came to power in 1997 determined to *save the NHS* but relatively soon found that, in an expression very popular at the time in Government, the levers in Whitehall weren't connected up and however hard you pulled on them nothing happened at the front line. Their frustration led them into a set of policies that both centralised and de-centralised at the same time.

They centralised to gain control of this rather anarchic situation. This took what at first sight seems a rather paradoxical form. It involved de-politicising the NHS. Many authorities were abolished and Ministers gave up their right to appoint members to those that remained. This resulted in more commercial style Boards where the non-executive members were appointed by the independent Appointments Commission on the basis of what they could bring to the Board and ignored political considerations altogether. This removal of the Secretary of State's power of patronage increased his power of management and direction. He no longer had to take any local political considerations into account in making directions but could begin to treat the Boards as subsidiaries of the national body.

This increase in power was reinforced, again seemingly paradoxically, by removing the direct link that had been there between the members or non-executives of Boards with the Secretary of State. Under previous regimes the Chairs of Authorities had direct access to the Secretary of State and could in effect bypass and sometimes undermine normal management processes by appealing to him or her over the heads of the managers and administrators in the system. The new arrangements saw the Boards fully accountable to the Chief Executive.

This de-politicisation strengthened the direct management line which was further reinforced when the posts of Permanent Secretary of the Department of Health and NHS Chief Executive were merged with my appointment in 2000. At the same time the NHS Plan brought with it national targets and national frameworks and all the other trappings of a single organisation.

By contrast, the establishment of NICE and CHI as independent bodies reduced the Secretary of State's powers but it also removed two major problems. No longer would the Secretary of State have to decide whether the NHS would pay for a particular therapy or be directly involved in criticising a hospital. There were now independent authorities for this. The Secretary of State had more freedom of action.

This centralisation gave the Secretary of State and the Chief Executive real power of action. It had de-politicised the intermediate layers and concentrated political and managerial power at the top. It attracted some criticism and complaints about the NHS lacking "democratic legitimacy" by removing the local political interests but these were dismissed at the time in the rush to save the NHS. We were all in a hurry and now had levers that were connected up …

The NHS centralised whilst at the same time in the NHS Plan stressing the importance of decentralisation as a means of getting greater local ownership and liberating front line creativity. There is an important point here. Any organisation needs a clearly defined centre and framework of roles and rules within which to decentralise. If there isn't a strong centre the operating units work entirely to their own agenda and any sense of an organisation moving in a shared direction with cooperation and sharing between its parts is lost. This is what the NHS had been like beforehand. The roles of both the centre and the units – and the linkages between the parts of the organisation – need to be clearly understood in an effective organisation. Neither of these was clearly defined in the NHS at the time.

There was inherent tension and scope for great confusion in all this. I used to use a simple model to explain to people what was happening: we needed over time to move from an 80:20 top down model where decisions were made centrally to a 20:80 bottom up model with most of the power of action was at a local level. There would be a period of transition in between during which power shifted. Figure 5.2 illustrates this.

I estimated that for the NHS Plan the first period of strengthening the centre would be from roughly 2000 to 2002, the transition from top down to bottom up would last for at least five years from 2003 to 2008 and that we might achieve the bottom up model by the end of the NHS Plan period in 2009 or 2010. As the figure shows the transition would not be smooth and there would be many bumps and problems on the way.

I predicted that there would be times when in response to a national crisis like a bad winter we would re-centralise some power and the line would spike upwards. Equally, there would be times when we decentralised too much and too fast so that the organisation lost overall coherence and control. Just such an example occurred in 2006 when financial problems in too many organisations around the country created a national NHS deficit for the first time in years and we had to re-centralise rapidly to gain control.

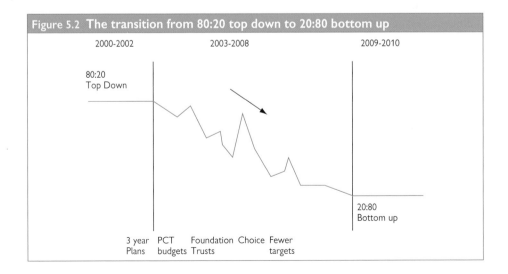

Figure 5.2 **The transition from 80:20 top down to 20:80 bottom up**

The whole process of decentralisation was complex and there were many milestones on the route. Five of these are shown along the bottom of Figure 5.2: creating three year budgets in 2001 gave NHS organisations more scope to plan; allocating most of the budget to PCTs from 2002 gave more local control; Foundation Trusts which were being created from 2002 had much greater autonomy; the introduction of greater patient choice promoted local responses; and the number of targets reduced as the main ones were achieved.

My predictions were very accurate about the journey itself. It was every bit as bumpy as I anticipated. I was, however, too optimistic that we would arrive at the 20:80 position within the NHS Plan period.

I used this figure very regularly with audiences throughout the NHS as a means of trying to show that we were serious about decentralising power and that, whilst there would be spikes upwards from time to time, the overall direction was consistent. It was part of my attempt to deal with the perception that we were talking about decentralising whilst hanging on to control.

This decentralisation trend was real. However, NHS organisations also found that the new organisations like NICE, CHI and the new Foundation Trust regulator, Monitor, all had some authority over them in the new arrangements. The power of the Department as a central controller may have reduced but there were other bodies that demanded attention.

Local freedom had real limitations and was tougher in many ways. Previously people could "delegate upwards" by saying that they couldn't deal with an issue locally. Sometimes this was true and sometimes it was a convenient excuse. Many people, however, relished the new freedom and the accountability: preferring to be in charge of their destiny as Chair or Chief Executive of a Foundation Trust Hospital to being, in effect, the manager of a subsidiary in an interfering group structure.

Decentralisation also attracted resistance. Three of the five milestones shown in Figure 5.1 – devolution to PCTs, the creation of Foundation Trusts, and patient choice – were unpopular with significant numbers of people. This meant that, whilst we tried to create an enabling environment, we often needed to apply pressure to make changes happen. Systems and people don't give up power readily and decentralisation takes power away from some people whilst giving it to others. We needed to keep the pace up.

I imagine that any reader with experience of management in other settings might ask why we made this all so complicated. Surely we should just set up a normal management structure and get on with delivering services: why did we need all this complexity? The truth is that in the NHS and other public structures of this kind we need to accommodate all these political as well as practical pressures and history always looms large. Even in the United States, home of private healthcare, I note there is enormous complexity in the regulations and limitations that surround healthcare and limit what might be seen as normal management processes in other organisations. Health is political.

I conceived of my objective as Chief Executive as steering my organisation as smoothly as possible down this line of transition whilst improving performance, delivering progressively more challenging targets and managing day to day events. It was not a straightforward task.

Whatever the next stages bring, the NHS has been on a long decentralisation journey. The original 1948 model had been akin to the nationalised industries set up at that period to run steel, coal mining and the railways. In thinking about its future we need to think much more in terms of systems than of organisations. Organograms will be less use to us than systems diagrams.

Demand side reforms – Primary Care Trusts: giving power to GPs

Primary Care Trusts (PCTs) were established in three waves from 2000 to take over many of the functions of Health Authorities and to work at the most local level in partnership with Local Authorities. It was the latest step in the long standing policy of promoting primary care and developing services in the community. Unlike the Primary Care Groups that had preceded them, PCTs had explicit authority and budgets. Alan Milburn asserted at their foundation that he wanted 80% of NHS funding to be allocated by PCTs. Very few budgets would be retained centrally and those only for professional education and training, research, major capital investment and service development and the more specialised services. Decision making about the services delivered locally should be made locally.

PCTs had three main roles. Firstly, they were charged with identifying the health needs of the population as a basis for what became known in NHS jargon as *commissioning* services to meet this need. Commissioning in the NHS in England meant and still means every aspect of this process: from the initial identification of need to the planning of services and the contractual arrangements with providers to deliver the appropriate services.

The creation of PCTs put financial decision making and planning alongside GPs in the community rather than alongside Consultants in hospitals. Representative GPs were given central roles in the internal leadership and management of PCTs. They were able to shape some of the demand for healthcare as well as the supply of services. As a result some priorities shifted towards the type of activity and problems that GPs routinely encountered in their surgeries. These were typically longer term conditions and things associated with mothers and young children on the one hand and older people on the other. They weren't the specialist conditions that so dominated hospitals.

The second role was in promoting public health. PCTs could link the activities needed to look after individuals with the activities designed to address the needs of the whole population. This process, in the best examples, brought together the expertise of public health doctors with that of primary care practitioners and led to many developments from greater focus on inequalities to the prescription of exercise and social activity as a means of promoting health and tackling long standing problems.

The third role, in developing primary care itself, gave scope for enormous creativity, particularly when it was associated with other improvements such as investment in premises and the development of new types of services such as Walk In Centres,

PCTs in some areas have performed very well in working with GPs and practice staff, local Trusts and clinicians, local authorities, voluntary organisations and others to improve health as well as services locally. Some, however, have become mired in bureaucracy, particularly around commissioning. If not handled imaginatively, this can degenerate into the worst sort of insurance scheme with rigid rules and an inability to respond to clinician creativity and patient need. This has alienated some GPs.

There has been another problem in their ability – and often inability – to make substantial change in secondary services. Powerful local hospitals can resist change successfully, particularly where it is seen to come from a local bureaucratic organisation. A final criticism has been that PCTs lack local democratic legitimacy as the local commissioners of services. Their accountability was through the NHS to Parliament. Their Board members, although local, were not appointed or elected locally. Even NHS Foundation Trusts had elected local Governors.

PCTs have shifted the balance of power a bit, but they have not transformed local services. They need further reform, with clinicians and local people – not just GPs or doctors – given a greater role. It remains to be seen how the proposed GP Commissioning Consortia will be configured in practice.

Demand side reform – offering patients choices

The other major change to the demand side was allowing patients to choose which hospitals and services they were referred to. This was intended to give patients more control and to encourage improvement and innovation in services as providers made themselves more responsive to patients' needs and wants.

Patients had always had some choices of services in the NHS. They could choose which GP to register with; although this was constrained by the availability of GPs locally and whether there was space on their lists. They could request a second opinion; although this was rarely taken up. Expectant mothers could choose their maternity unit; although choices were limited by availability of places. More popular units booked up faster. In addition patients could use any emergency services, although their condition might dictate they got as quickly as possible to the nearest hospital.

The new policy opened up choices for all aspects of elective outpatients and surgery. Patients would be able to choose where they were referred from, initially, a short list of local hospitals to, eventually, a list of any public or private provider in the country that met NHS standards and prices. A computer system *"Choose and Book"* was designed to support this based on the model of airline booking systems. You could book anywhere at a date that suited you, provided a seat/bed/clinic slot was available.

In practice take up by patients was slow in the early years as most patients chose to go to their local provider. There was, however, as we saw in Figure 4.6 at the end of the last chapter an immediate effect on NHS surgical providers when in April 2003 all patients who had been waiting more than 6 months for admission to hospital were offered a choice of going to other hospitals. The numbers waiting more than six months fell dramatically. I remember noticing this with satisfaction and investigating the reason. It emerged that Hospital Chief Executives had worked hard to eliminate over six month waiters so that their patients wouldn't be offered choice and go elsewhere. It was a rare example of a positive unintended consequence of a system change. They are generally the other way round.

This policy of choice has attracted a great deal of controversy and been much criticised. Some clinicians have, rightly, pointed out that the choice patients most want is to have treatment options explained by their clinician. They also want continuity of treatment and follow up. The clinician's fear was that greater patient choice over hospital might lead to fragmentation and sub-optimisation of care.

The issue here is about how this policy is implemented. It isn't an either/or situation. The choices of hospital need not mean fragmentation of services if it is managed well. The risk of this is far greater with long-term conditions, mental health, cancer and palliative care where continuity is important. It is less relevant for one-off events like cataracts, haemorrhoids and varicose veins. As a patient I would expect my clinician to advise me about this. As a policy maker I would expect PCTs and future GP Consortia to offer choices of packages of care – combined diagnosis, treatment, follow up – in the more complex cases where continuity is so crucial.

Why as a patient can I not have both sorts of choice, even if one is more important than the other? Why should I not choose to go to the NHS hospital Y not NHS hospital X for minor surgery, an endoscopy or an X ray? I understand that the clinical care will be the same but the people at Y are friendlier and I can get car parking. Why should I not decide to go the NHS hospital rather than the private one because I know there are plenty of back up services, *crash teams* and

Intensive Care Units if something goes wrong rather than the smart looking private hospital where emergency care is an ambulance ride away?

The biggest impact of choice has so far been on the behaviour of service providers. The threat of patients choosing to go to another hospital is real and has led to some improvements and innovations; although it is not a necessary or foregone conclusion. As in other policies the key is how it is implemented and how the downsides or risks – which always exist with any policy – are managed.

It has also been argued that only the articulate middle classes would benefit from exercising choice and as a result would have another lever to ensure that they got all the best services. Moreover, there was the risk that unpopular hospitals and services in poorer areas would lose patients to wealthier ones and, once again, the poorest and neediest would lose out.

These again are real risks; but they, again, can be identified and managed. PCTs and GP Consortia can commission services to counteract this. The most important point is that risks must be identified and understood and opportunities created for the more disadvantaged to exercise their own choices. It is noticeable in London that some hospitals are more popular than others with different ethnic groups. These hospitals are better able to meet their needs for appropriate birthing and death and offer space for their own rituals and customs. This is a profoundly important aspect of being responsive to patients as a community and an example of people exercising choice.

Patient choice became a highly symbolic policy and a dividing line between those who believed in a market and those who wanted planned services. The truth – that choice could be useful but the downsides needed to be managed and that it was helping shift the culture to become more patient centred – became irrelevant. Its proponents talked it up as being a major leap forward in patient control. The opposition to it also held more than a hint of old fashioned paternalism and professional protectionism. These two aspects came together for me late one evening in a traditional London Club where I was confronted by an *Old Labour Peer*.

He was a man I knew of with a long and distinguished record of standing up for the working classes and was very much a man of the people. He was shocked by the whole idea of patient choice. *"Nigel,"* he said, *"You and I know that some doctors are better than others but the danger in this policy is that we mustn't say that in public because it will undermine trust in doctors and we can't have that."* I was deeply shocked in my turn.

It gave me at the time a startling insight into the mindset of some of those opposed to patient choice. It also offered a vivid glimpse of the fight inside the Labour Party over these reforms.

Supply side reforms – NHS Foundation Trusts

On the supply side NHS Foundation Trusts, like PCTs, were also in part the product of NHS history. There had been a long held policy of giving more management control to operating units with the introduction of General Managers in 1985 following the Griffiths Review and the creation of NHS Trusts from 1991.[6]

In the event NHS Trusts had proved to have relatively few freedoms. Many ideas to strengthen their freedoms or create new bodies were proposed. I recall as the Chief Executive of the Oxford Radcliffe visiting the Treasury in 1996 with a Director from Rothschild's to put forward the proposal that hospitals like mine should be able to opt out of direct control and become mutual organisations owned by their patients, staff and referring hospitals and GPs. We were politely received. The idea was toyed with but a General Election was only a year away and there was no political will and energy in a dying Government to do anything with it.

These sorts of ideas, both from the UK and abroad, were once again discussed at the time of the NHS Plan and crystallised out into the policy to create Foundation Trusts in 2002.[7] Hospitals and NHS service providers were mostly NHS Trusts at the time – organisations which had a degree of autonomy from their immediate Health Authorities but which were accountable to me as the NHS Chief Executive. Their Chief Executives and Boards had long complained about their limited freedoms and the way in which Ministers and the Chief Executive could intervene in their activity at any point without needing any more legal justification than that, in effect, they judged it necessary.

NHS Foundation Trusts, on the other hand, were to have their freedoms established in law. Ministers and the Chief Executive would only have limited powers over them and, instead of accountability to the centre, they would be accountable to their own local Board of Governors and regulated by a new NHS Foundation Trust regulator. This regulator, Monitor, would be responsible for scrutinising their business plans and imposing appropriate measures where necessary to ensure that they remained viable for the long term. It would also be responsible for considering a Trust's bid to become a Foundation Trust and authorising – or not – their transition. Monitor, unlike the Department, had no direct management responsibility for them and would not be engaged in any policy issues.

The establishment of Foundation Trusts was also highly controversial and became the subject of very hotly contested debates in Parliament. There were fears that this represented a step towards privatisation of the hospitals and clearing the way to sell off NHS assets to the private sector at a later date. Other critics, who didn't go that far, nevertheless saw it as breaking up the unity of the NHS, fragmenting planning and introducing destructive competition in which

Foundation Trusts would maximise their position at the expense of the whole system.

There was also opposition from the Treasury which saw this policy of giving Trusts greater autonomy as dangerously increasing financial risk in the NHS. Such bodies would not be controlled by the Department of Health – which, in any case, they viewed with the suspicion with which they regarded all spending Departments. They could at least attempt to control the Department through the links that bound Government together at the centre and through the Public Service Agreements. The Foundation Trusts, however, would be right outside their power and left in the hands of an independent regulator. They didn't like it.

Worse still the Department was proposing to give the Foundation Trusts extensive borrowing powers which, if exercised, would add to the public sector debt and therefore to the Public Sector Borrowing Requirement (PSBR) which the Treasury was committed to controlling as one of the central planks of economic strategy. All this was seen as very high risk.

This was the source of one of the most significant internal government battles about health of this period. Alan Milburn was adamant that his plans must stand. The Chancellor was equally immovable. The issues were argued long and hard in separate sessions by the politicians, by their political advisers and by officials. We argued over figures and assessments of risk; but the real battle was political. Was the Government prepared to decentralise and trust local people to take responsibility or was it unwilling to take that risk even though it might bring significant benefit?

The battle was symbolic of the Government's internal struggles about the future direction of public services. Alan Milburn showed that, unlike many Cabinet colleagues, he was prepared to take on the Chancellor and not give way. It was from this period that he was seen as an ultra-Blairite: promoting the Prime Minister's liberalising, market orientated and reforming vision as against the more centralist and controlling policies favoured by Gordon Brown. It was a tension at the heart of the Government.

In the end there was a compromise. Foundation Trusts retained more freedoms than the Treasury wanted but borrowing was heavily constrained and the PSBR was safe from this source of risk.

Supply side reform – opening the market to the private sector

The second great supply side reform was allowing the private sector to provide services for NHS patients. This started, as I have already described, as a temporary measure designed to take the pressure off the NHS as it struggled to increase activity levels and deliver waiting list reductions. Restrictions were lifted so that local NHS organisations – PCTs or Trusts – could contract with non-NHS organisations to provide services.

At the same time, however, the Department set out to tender for private sector organisations to establish so-called Independent Sector Diagnostic and Treatment Centres (ISTCs) which would be new or re-designed units able to deliver a small range of high volume services such as day case surgery, scans or diagnostic scoping. They would operate without all the overheads of the big NHS hospitals.

The two approaches were very different. The first allowed local NHS organisations to control the services delivered privately. Trusts might buy in extra capacity to support their work. The second, however, was nationally driven and, whilst directed towards needs identified by local PCTs, introduced new providers into a locality in competition with existing ones. This naturally produced tension and conflict.

There were many issues to deal with. Which patients would go to ISTCs and which to the NHS? Would the ISTCs *cream off* the easy cases, maximising their profits and leaving all the complex patients to the NHS? What subsidy would they have to receive to compensate for only having short term three year contracts? Would all the same quality standards apply? Would NHS doctors and other staff be able to work in the ISTCs in their own time? If not, where would the staffing come from? Who would handle any follow-ups and long term complications? Procuring these services would be a complex business which would involve both a great deal of technical detail and the careful management of local medical and NHS interests, some of which strongly opposed the introduction of new entrants into the local health system.

The NHS and the Department contained very few people with any substantial amount of private sector experience. Similarly commercial organisations had little experience of public bodies or public service. The result, as I had observed over many years, was that both parties were frustrated by their dealings with the other. I heard private sector people talk of the difficulty of doing business with the NHS and the NHS describe how private sector organisations didn't understand what was needed. It was as if they were talking different languages.

We set up a Commercial Advisory Board in the Department to help bridge the communication gap and offer advice to all sides. Sir William Wells, a long term NHS Non Executive with extensive commercial experience, chaired it and he appointed an excellent group from a variety of different commercial backgrounds who offered their services to us for free. It worked well in those early days in raising awareness in both sectors of the needs of the other; but later with a change of Prime Minister the political climate hardened against the private sector and in September 2007 the Commercial Advisory Board resigned in protest at the changed environment.

We needed some new people and new skills in the Department to manage the procurement. Ken Anderson was appointed to do so and to head up the wider work on the engagement of the private sector as the NHS's first Commercial Director. He in turn brought in a team of people from different disciplines and backgrounds to handle the detail.

Anderson's team could not as London based newcomers to the NHS deal with the relationships with the local health systems. This fell largely to John Bacon as Delivery Director General and his team. I made it clear that I expected Chief Executives locally – PCTs, Trusts and Strategic Health Authorities – to work together on this as NHS leaders and that the Commercial and Delivery teams centrally would do the same. This was simple to say but the truth was that these changes were very divisive both locally and nationally.

There were several aspects to this. Many Chief Executives could see that their own organisations would be adversely affected; they had some of their clinicians up in arms and, in some cases, had strong personal reservations about involving the private sector. Nationally the Commercial team, like any new group, were anxious to establish themselves and approached their work with a very different style to the people they had to work with. They had the advantage and disadvantage of having a high profile politically. They were in and out of Ministers' offices and on occasion fell into the familiar trap which can affect anyone working too closely with power of both being seduced by it and behaving as if they themselves possessed it. The longer serving civil servants were less susceptible to this as they had been brought up on the motto of *"Speak truth unto power"* and knew that all personal power is transitory …

Ministers as one would expect preferred the newcomers.

Gradually and without fanfare the policy changed. The tendering for ISTCs marked a new phase in policy in which an element of private sector competition was to become a permanent part of NHS delivery and not just a temporary expedient. The argument was that we needed to maintain a sufficient level of external challenge to keep the NHS on its toes. The private sector needed to be able to bid for enough work to be sustainable in the longer run. A one-off contract wouldn't serve this purpose so we had further waves of procurement for ISTCs and the expansion of the choices offered to patients so that they always involved at least one private sector option.

I well remember several occasions when my colleagues nationally and locally let me know about the problems and the tensions that private sector involvement was causing. Why, I was asked by some, was I encouraging private competition just when the NHS was improving and starting to deliver on its targets? My answer, no doubt unconvincing to many, was that private sector competition would help us improve even faster. It is to the enormous credit of all those NHS and

Department leaders that, despite the tensions and some hard words, they held the service together and continued to deliver improvements.

A lot of this, however, was an uphill struggle. Most NHS staff and members of the public thought of the NHS in terms of the actual bricks and mortar of the hospitals and expected care to be given by NHS employed staff in NHS owned facilities. In the Department however we were at this stage starting to think of the NHS as more like a guarantee or a promise of care. The NHS would make sure you were looked after well and got the care you needed whether you were treated in an NHS Hospital or a charity or private one. You would be an NHS patient in every case and entitled to the same standards, rights and privileges and you would access it in the same way through your GP, phone line or Accident and Emergency Department.

Thinking of the NHS in this way – *re-conceptualising* it in the jargon – opened up enormous possibilities for innovative services. We were no longer bound by old restrictions as to who might offer a service or how. We were, however, as tightly bound as ever by the vision and values of the NHS. This was not an insurance system, although some people began to talk as if it was. The NHS remained a social contract not a commercial one. Funding would continue to come from taxes and services would continue to be available to every citizen according to their need and regardless of their ability to pay. The NHS would continue to be free at the point of need but there would be greater flexibility in the way in which it was delivered.

There was a big problem however, which John Bacon was the first to spot. By late 2003 we had sufficient capacity in the NHS. We were reducing waiting times and the numbers on the waiting list consistently month by month. We didn't need extra capacity from the private sector. This was excellent news but it also gave us a difficulty. Put simply it confronted us with the fact that if we kept on introducing private sector competition there would inevitably be some reduction in NHS activity – it was a zero sum game – and that would mean both that some NHS facilities might have to close and that some of the new developments in the pipeline would not be needed.

The choices were obvious: we could keep on with our policy of opening the market and accept the consequences to the NHS or we could drop it. We ended up trying to compromise.

This was the point of greatest tension between me and my managerial and civil servant colleagues and the politicians and their aides. It was interesting that a lot of people didn't want to hear John's analysis. I remember one economist looking at the graphs I was showing him of activity levels and waiting list falls and seeking to disprove them. He couldn't. Another Number 10 adviser told me that it was irrelevant because the key thing was to get the private sector involved. Others ducked the issue.

Part of the problem was that the policy had been introduced by saying that the private sector was here to support the NHS with extra capacity but now we could see that it would damage some NHS organisations. Another part was that the modernisers of New Labour in the Department of Health and Number 10 were well ahead of the mainstream of the Labour Party which was still coming to terms with Foundation Trusts, patient choice and using the private sector at all. The politicians had very little room to manoeuvre.

From time to time ministers were pressed to say how much of NHS activity would be provided by the private sector. They settled at this stage on the figure of no more than 15%. By 2009 when the reforming edge had gone the then Secretary of State, Andy Burnham said that the NHS would be the *"preferred provider"* of services and downplayed the private sector contribution altogether.

It all got very difficult. Leaders in the NHS could see clearly what was happening. They knew that there would need to be closures and cancellation of development projects. Their complaints were seen by some of the politicians as evidence that they were anti-reform and purely self interested. It was seen as the NHS being unwilling to change. They, in turn, saw the politicians as being unwilling to face up to reality and, even, being duplicitous. The upshot of all this was some mutual loss of confidence and a lack of clear explanations about the policy being give both to the public and the NHS. I, John Bacon and others were caught in the middle of this trying to steer the best path we could.

This was the clearest example in my time as Chief Executive of political differences within the party of Government spilling over into policy making in a destructive way. The differences prevented us from making a clear and timely decision on a pressing issue with the result that it had to be dealt with later in a more rushed and unsatisfactory way.

I suspect that there is nothing unusual, special or even odd about the UK in this regard. Some countries, like China and South Africa, have very obviously parallel party processes behind the scenes where policy differences are or aren't thrashed out before policies are promulgated by the Minister in public. In other countries, like the United States, it is the special interests and lobby groups, many of them commercial, which most obviously influence policy in this way. Greater transparency is needed in either system.

My own view as Chief Executive was that the policy was important and worthwhile. I wanted to see more challenge in the system as a spur to innovation. I wanted the private sector working in the NHS on our terms and within our overall goals to achieve equity as well as excellence and efficiency.

The policy continued. Many people have now been treated as NHS patients in private sector facilities; although it is far less than the 15% limit. We didn't however take any significant action to reduce NHS expansion at the time with the result that over-capacity contributed to later financial problems. This led to the necessary reductions in NHS activities and capacity being made in a relatively rushed and unplanned way some time after John had pointed out the problem.

Transactional reforms – money following patients

Several years earlier the Conservative administration which introduced the separation of purchasers and providers coined the expression "*money following patients*" to describe how Trusts which attracted more contracts from their purchasers would receive more money. Successful and popular hospitals and other services would benefit. It only had limited success because contracts weren't legally binding and contract pricing was often not directly related to the number of patients.

This changed with the introduction of legally binding contracts and a national tariff for pricing. Money really would follow patients under this "*payment by results*" (PBR) scheme. This was another major change to the system which had the potential to change behaviours and patterns of service.

There was a well recognised problem that providers are only paid for certain sorts of activity: so called *Finished Consultant Episodes* (FCEs) – essentially completed hospital admissions under a Consultant; outpatient attendances and certain categories of tests. They provided many other services. Moreover there was no way of paying for many desirable innovations and improvements in services such as telephone consultations; home intervention teams and the added value of "*one stop shops*".

It is well known in any country which attempts to link pay to specific activities that the definition of the activity – what is actually measured and attracts the money – determines what gets done. In insurance systems in particular this can lead to endless arguments for patients about whether specific activities are covered.

PBR had the potential to make the situation better. It could introduce much greater flexibility into the payment system so that providers really did get paid for what they did that benefited patients. It could also incentivise desirable activities by, for example, paying proportionately more for community based alternatives to hospital admissions or for day surgery rather than inpatient surgery.

PBR takes a long time to implement fully and satisfactorily. In the early years it could make matters worse by only identifying a narrow range of prices. It might not distinguish, for example, between a child's relatively routine admission to a general hospital and a worse case of the same condition admitted to a specialised unit. This latter case might well be a better but much more expensive option. An inadequate payment system would fail to incentivise and reward the best behaviour.

During my time as Chief Executive PBR was in its infancy. My colleagues tried to manage its introduction sensibly and flexibly so as to minimise the down sides. Five years later it has become much more sophisticated but is still being developed.

System reforms – regulation and quality

These reforms also required us to change the wider environment within which NHS organisations and their partners in social care worked. In line with our policy of decentralisation we moved from a directly managed system where the Department provided all the guidance and control to a regulated one where organisations independent of the Department set standards, offered guidance and inspected and regulated. Our two main goals – the principles that guided our behaviour – were to create an environment which promoted quality throughout the system and to make sure that it was properly regulated.

By 2000, as described in Chapter 3, we already had a number of important organisations within the field of quality. There was NICE, designed to review new therapies and promote clinical guidelines and The Commission for Health Improvement (CHI) and the Social Services Inspectorate (SSI) to inspect and quality assure in health and social services respectively. In 2001 we created the Modernisation Agency to promote quality improvement as was discussed at some length in the last chapter. From 2001 onwards we added the National Patient Safety Agency, the National Clinical Assessment Authority and others to provide more specific leadership in these areas and we agreed a Standards Framework to guide the work of all these bodies.

These bodies changed and developed their operations over the years with, for example, CHI becoming CHAI (the Commission for Healthcare Audit and Inspection – known as the Healthcare Commission) in 2004 and merging with the parts of SSI which covered adult social care in 2009 to form the Care Quality Commission (CQC). Throughout this process it acquired new and more wide ranging powers of regulation as well as inspection. Similarly the Modernisation Agency became the National Institute for Innovation and Improvement in 2005 as discussed in the last chapter.

The health sector already had a number of long standing and more recent regulators charged with oversight of particular areas which included, for example, The General Medical Council established following the Medical Act of 1858 (the first regulation of doctors was in a Parliamentary Statute of 1511) and the Human Fertilisation and Embryology Authority created following the 1990 Human Fertilisation and Embryology Act.

There were some simplifications of these regulatory systems during this period. The most significant addition was with the creation of Monitor in January 2004 to authorise and regulate NHS Foundation Trusts. It is independent of central government and directly accountable to Parliament for approving Foundation

Trusts, ensuring they meet their licence conditions and supporting their development.

This shortened version of the full list of national bodies which were designed variously to support and regulate the NHS and the health sector gives a glimpse into the complexity of this area. It explains why Chief Executives and NHS Boards were always so concerned about the number of organisations which had rights of inspection over them.

From time to time the Department has reviewed and reduced numbers with, for example, the Arms Length Body Review which reported in 2004 reducing numbers from 38 to 20 with a planned saving of £500 million.[8] Such bodies tend to grow over time as politics and the public demand new safety nets. As part of this cycle there are regular "bonfires of the quangos". A new Arms Length Body Review set up in 2010 is making similar reductions.

Managing the reform

In the last chapter I described the way in which we managed service improvements through a combination of quality improvements methodologies and performance management. This chapter has described how at the same time we introduced a whole series of fundamental system reforms. There is more to come. In the next chapters we will deal with changes in staff pay and conditions, the introduction of new technology, changed relationships with patients and new approaches to health promotion – all of this being undertaken in the same time frame.

The leadership and management task was immensely complex. Each individual issue needed attention whilst the whole package required balance and integration. It became more complicated where there was tension and conflict as there was over the opening of the market to the private sector.

It was here that I believe the "Top Team" came into its own. Every month I brought together for a day the Chief Executives of the 28 Strategic Health Authorities with my national Directors and the National Clinical Directors or Czars. It was a working meeting. We surfaced and argued out the issues. I made clear which the non-negotiable items on the current agenda were, they made clear where their sticking points were and together we worked for agreement on the rest. From time to time we invited Ministers or even the Prime Minister to join us, enabling us to question policy and feed back directly from the NHS; but it was primarily a management meeting.

The challenge for us as the leadership of the NHS and the implementers of the NHS Plan was to craft the best way forward through all this complexity. We were able to do it very effectively from 2002 to 2005 largely through the development of relationships, shared endeavour and a shared commitment to the NHS. About a third of our members were clinicians, a further third had a technical background of some sort and about a third were, like me, generalists.

My task was to make this team work effectively together and to ensure that they were able to transmit the core messages and agreements to and from their own people locally. Each of the others had their own teams to lead and the SHA Chief Executives in particular had an important role in bringing together their 30 or so Chief Executives and Directors in some sort of local leadership group once a month.

These arrangements meant that the 1,200 or so people who occupied the most senior executive leadership positions in the NHS came together around the same agenda every month; each of them only one step away from me as Chief Executive of the whole NHS. It was what I called this *"Community of Chief Executives"* which held us together through these times and which I will discuss in more detail alongside other aspects of leadership in Chapter 9.

Conclusions and key points

1. Reform and re-design of the system can bring big benefits. However, these sorts of reforms – involving such radical changes as introducing private sector provision into a state system – are of intense public and political interest and can't be handled by clinicians and managers alone.

2. In the UK as we moved from essentially a nationalised industry approach to healthcare to a national health system which made use of other providers we came up against political, public and staff opposition. We were dealing with some issues which had helped define the NHS since its inception in 1948. It was about symbolism as well as practical reality.

3. Decentralisation brings benefits but needs to take place within a clear national framework and may require the initial strengthening of the centre so that subsequent decentralisation is coherent and effective. We planned to move from an 80:20 top down approach to a 20:80 bottom up one but recognised this would not be a smooth progression from one to the other.

4. Decentralisation shifts power from one group to another and will inevitably be opposed to some extent by the losers. It therefore needs to be led and implemented firmly. It also requires a new framework to secure quality and appropriate regulation.

5. Offering patients more choice made relatively little impact initially on their behaviour but it did affect the way NHS organisations reacted and thereby created some significant improvements. It also revealed some deep seated paternalistic and, even, protectionist attitudes amongst professionals and policy makers.

Conclusions and key points (*Continued*)

6. Whilst private sector providers were initially introduced into the NHS to create additional capacity they were retained to provide continued competition. However, the extent of their involvement was limited and they operated within the overall NHS framework.

7. All these changes had a cost. Expansion of the private sector meant reductions in NHS capacity and activity. These costs needed to be anticipated and actively managed. However, political considerations made it hard to do this with the result that problems were stored up for the future.

8. The radical nature and the number of changes tested both the unity of the NHS and the relationship between politicians and executives. It was very important to have good mechanisms – like the Top Team – for ensuring that the whole of the senior leadership were able to participate in decision making and be willing to buy in to the whole process and its consequences.

9. Improvement had to be maintained **and** it had to be publicised to ensure momentum and show that the NHS could improve and was improving.

References

1. Department of Health (2000) *The NHS Plan – a Plan for investment, a Plan for reform*, July, p 96.
2. Department of Health (2002) *Delivering the NHS Plan: next steps for investment, next steps for reform*; CM5503, 18 April.
3. Department of Health (2004) *The NHS Improvement Plan – putting people at the heart of public services*; CM 6268, 24 June.
4. Cabinet Office (2006) *The UK Government's Approach to Public Sector Reform*.
5. Edwards B, Fall M (2005) *The Executive years of the NHS: the England account 1985–2003*; Nuffield Trust, 14 Sept.
6. Ibid.
7. Department of Health (2002) *Delivering the NHS Plan*; CM 5503 18 April.
8. *Arms Length Body Review*, 22 July 2004, Department of Health.

Chapter 6

The NHS workforce

"*It simply isn't legal*", the Medical Director of the hospital on the edge of London assured me. "*Nurses are not allowed to order X rays. It's against the law.*" It didn't matter that I told him that there were nurses in the A and E Department of his neighbouring hospital who did just that. He was quite adamant. They were breaking the law.

We looked at each other in mutual incomprehension. It was a Friday afternoon and I was visiting a number of NHS facilities in the area, meeting staff, answering their questions and seeing for myself what the problems were and what people were doing about them. I had just come from the hospital in the next Borough where I had been interested to see that the Consultants and nurses in the busy A and E Department had decided to give the more senior nurses the right to order X rays for patients who fitted certain protocols.

It was a well thought through and organised practice which cut out a step in the normal process. An experienced nurse was able to order an X ray for a patient so that they had it with them when they saw the doctor rather than first having to see the doctor, then get the X ray and then see the doctor again. It was all very logical, safe and appropriate and of course legal …

The Medical Director had just been telling me about how hard pressed the A and E was. I asked him if allowing some of the nurses to order X rays or other tests might speed things up. He wouldn't hear of it: not while he was Medical Director he told me; adding rather pompously that he wasn't going to take responsibility for breaking the law.

It was the sort of situation I was to encounter many times in the NHS where there was a casual assumption that a traditional practice was the way things had to be and that alternatives if not actually illegal were certainly unsafe and even unethical. It was an attitude that supported a rigid demarcation in roles and allowed for little flexibility of operation. In due course the Modernisation Agency approach with its "process mapping", PDSA cycles and other methods of service re-design would bring about massive changes in A and E as we saw in Chapter 4.

Re-designing jobs and restructuring the health workforce was a crucial part of implementing the NHS Plan.

The human resources strategy

The *HR in the NHS Plan* published in July 2002 described the notion of the "*skills escalator*". It had two parts. Firstly, anyone who joined the NHS could progress through it picking up skills and professional qualifications as appropriate with their opportunities and their pay reflecting their performance at every stage. The second part was that as the environment changed and jobs were re-designed, particular tasks and roles could move down the organisation and be done by people with lower levels of skills and experience just as safely provided appropriate training, supervision and other systems were in place. It required "*an integrated approach to modernising pay, learning and development, regulation and workforce planning.*"[1]

I will concentrate here only on the two major elements that were the focus of the most effort across the NHS: restructuring and re-design of jobs and the negotiation and implementation of new pay and conditions. I am conscious that this ignores some very important areas.

The NHS Plan called for expansion of staffing. At the time unemployment was low and there were more vacancies than applicants and many of our policies were therefore about recruiting and retaining people. This included a major back-to-nursing campaign to attract back women who had left to have children with retraining available as well as a package of benefits including "term time" contracts and "family friendly" hours.

Regulatory arrangements were outdated and didn't reflect modern practices or encourage change. The profile and skill base of human resources management needed to be raised. A great deal of effort was also put into increasing levels of education and training – including the opening of three new medical schools – and promoting innovation in content and design. At the end of the period a re-structuring of medical training through Modernising Medical Careers began.

External issues also intruded into the NHS with, for example, a major rise in national insurance adding costs. More importantly, the NHS had to deal with the European Working Time Directive which limited the number of hours staff could work and particularly affected doctors' rotas. It had massive knock on effects. In the best cases this led to redesign of services and breaking down of demarcations as rotas were combined and nurses took on more roles. In the worst cases Trusts simple spent more money to prop up unreformed rotas and used more locums. It provided yet another reason why service and job design needed to be undertaken together.

We start here, however, with the most radical area of re-structuring and will move on via staff numbers to look at staff contracts.

Restructuring the workforce

As services are re-designed and systems change – and, crucially, as technology advances – there are needs for many different roles and, of course, the elimination of some. More than 60% of NHS expenditure is spent on paying people. How the NHS deploys and develops these people is therefore vital both in terms of quality and expenditure.

There are conflicting pressures here. There is a long established trend in health systems generally towards more extensive training, tighter professional barriers and greater specialisation in order to improve patient care. This has been one of the factors leading to improved healthcare around the world. Professor Sir Brian Jarman and colleagues' study of 1999 showed, for example, that in English acute hospitals the number of doctors had an inverse correlation with death rates.[2] In other words the more doctors there were in the hospital the lower the death rate.

However, most healthcare is now delivered outside hospitals and is not about life or death. Research shows that looking across a country as a whole – and not just at hospitals – lower mortality rates are correlated with numbers of primary care doctors and not with the numbers of hospital specialists.[3] Other research undertaken in the UK and abroad has shown that health workers other than doctors may be as effective at certain clinical procedures and may be preferred by some patients.[4] Taken together this research points to the need for more primary care doctors and to the scope of other practitioners, under the right circumstances, taking on work previously done by doctors.

Some changes to roles were strongly supported by doctors. I recall being lobbied by Palliative Care physicians who wanted their nursing colleagues to be able to prescribe opiates to patients under strict protocols. They argued that it was absurd that experienced nurses had to find a doctor, sometimes in the middle of the night, to sign routine scripts as their patients deteriorated. It was not only an irritant for the professionals they argued, but delayed much needed pain relief for their patients.

Many such changes, however, were opposed by the professional bodies, jealous of their members' rights and keen to maintain control over tasks that only they could do. It is, of course, absolutely right that the scope of practice should be controlled and that clinical tasks should only be undertaken by people properly trained and qualified for the task. Regulation has a critical role in healthcare. However, it is also important that traditional practices – or demarcations – do not get in the way of people becoming properly trained and qualified in new tasks if it is appropriate for them to do so.

Over time negotiation, perseverance and hard work on the details of protocols and practice have brought changes. Nurse Consultants and nurse practitioners with expanded roles were created as were nurse endoscopists and other specialist nurses. Senior nurses and other senior members of the professions allied to medicine were given limited prescribing rights after appropriate training and imaging technicians, physiotherapy assistants and others were able to take on wider roles under the supervision of fully qualified professionals.

There may have been opposition from the professional bodies but many individuals led by example. I was exposed to these issues early in my time in Oxford when two young trauma surgeons, Keith Willett and Peter Worlock, asked for my support in redesigning their service. They told me that, given the importance of the "golden hour" after an accident, it was essential to have a Trauma Consultant in the hospital at all times to treat patients immediately on their arrival. They therefore proposed that they and the other Consultants working in the service would do 24 hour shifts during which they would stay in the hospital at all times.

They recognised that this would have profound knock on effects on the rest of the service and had worked through how other roles would have to change with nurses taking on some things previously done by doctors. Radically they insisted that only nurses could discharge patients from the wards – as they would be the ones offering continuity of care and observation of the patients – and they created a new group of trauma technicians to take on some duties previously done by doctors and nurses. They had costed out the changes in staffing that would be necessary to make it self-funding and re-organised the training rotas so that trainees gained a better experience. They had even set up a research programme which would look at the affect on them and their families as well as on the service provided to patients.

It was a Chief Executive's dream: a fully thought through proposal which improved quality without additional cost. The medical profession's representatives hated it. They feared it would be a bridgehead from which management would insist that all Consultants spent nights in the hospital and they resented the increased responsibility for the nurses. I remember how the representative of the Royal College of Surgeons who sat on the interview panel tried to put candidates off the new Consultant posts that were needed. He failed. The young bright Consultants we appointed in 1994 were incredibly enthusiastic to be part of this visionary service which they saw as being the way of the future. They are still there 16 years later.

Staff numbers

The NHS more than achieved its targeted increase in staff numbers. All sectors of the workforce expanded. In the 10 year period from the end of 1999 to the end of 2009, the period covered by the NHS Plan, the total workforce increased by almost a third or 304,000 in Full Time Equivalents. [*]

---

[*] The increase in the actual number of extra individuals, the headcount – including part time staff – was 333,648. I have used Full Time Equivalent here and elsewhere in this chapter as more accurately representing workforce capacity. *NHS Staffing Overview 2009*: NHS Information Centre, 25 March 2010.

This was very welcome because there were severe shortages in some areas. However, the NHS came under great pressure from staff and Ministers to recruit very quickly – this was a popular policy with the public and showed the new money was bringing tangible results – and in retrospect we can see that it was too fast. In this pressurised rush for delivery some Trusts hit the targets without using the opportunity to redesign services and roles. It was a wasted opportunity.

Figure 6.1 shows the relative proportions of staff groups in the NHS in September 2005 with about half being professionally qualified, another third working in direct support of clinical staff and the remaining sixth engaged in the infrastructure – from estates, catering and IT to finance, human resources and management.

These figures show that the number of managers in the NHS was less than 3% of total staffing. This was, however, the area which saw the greatest increase proportionally from 23,378 in 1999 to 42,509 in 2009 or 6% a year as the NHS moved to becoming a more managed service. In absolute terms of course this increase of 19,000 is far less than the increase of 75,000 nurses, 44,000 doctors and 41,000 professional scientists, therapists and technicians.[5]

The professionally qualified groups still dominated the numbers and the increases. They accounted for more than half of the overall increase in staffing with a rise of 163,000, including, 44,000 doctors; the clinical support functions contributed about a quarter with growth of 75,000; and the central functions represented about a fifth of the overall increase or 61,000.[6]

Given our emphasis on job redesign we might have expected less growth in the professionals and more in the other groups. The explanation seems to be that because the UK employed proportionately less doctors than most other comparable countries – although it had a similar proportion of nurses – there was a case to increase the number of doctors as part of the "catch up" recommended by Derek Wanless. Table 6.2 shows how the proportions changed.

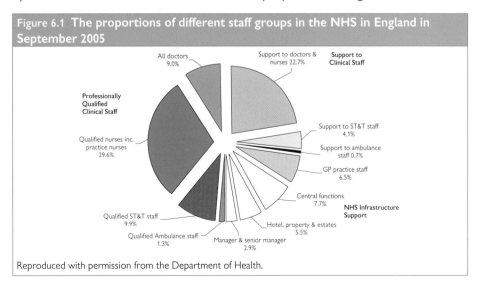

Figure 6.1 **The proportions of different staff groups in the NHS in England in September 2005**

Reproduced with permission from the Department of Health.

Whatever the merit of the catch-up argument, we were not as radical in role redesign as we were in service redesign and system reform. There is much more that could be done here.

It may be that financial considerations will lead to the necessary changes whether directly or by stealth. However, there is another option. Professor Willett and colleagues were able to make change in Oxford because they were dealing with their own services and were not external managers introducing or imposing change. Meanwhile GPs have quietly led the largest restructuring of the workforce in the NHS – and possibly in any health system in the world – within their own practices. A service that was very largely delivered by the doctors themselves at the end of the last century has become one where many different groups – nurses, therapists and counselors – provide large parts of it, often with enhanced value.

GPs have also changed the nature of their own role more profoundly and opened up a gap between partners and others. The workforce figures show that the biggest percentage increase in staffing numbers between 2000 and 2009 was in "other GPs" – fully qualified GPs who were not partners in practices. This went up from 786 in 2000 to 8,304 in 2009 or by practically 10,000%.[7]

Traditionally, GPs have been self-employed partners in a practice and have a service contract, not an employment contract, with the NHS locally. Since changes to their contracts in 2003 made it easier – and profitable to do so - they have started to employ other GPs on salaries rather than make them partners. From 2003 onwards half all new GPs have been salaried and the trend is increasing. In the year to September 2009 there were 266 new partners in GP practices but 1,641 new salaried GPs.[8]

There is a history to this. I remember in the 1990s trying to persuade GP practices in London to recruit salaried GPs in areas where populations were generally under-served by doctors and where it was difficult to get GPs willing to

Table 6.1 **Number of doctors and nurses per 1,000 in the population in the UK, France and Germany 2000 to 2008**				
	Doctors/1,000 in 2000	Doctors/1,000 in 2008	Nurses/1,000 in 2000	Nurses/1,000 in 2008
UK	1.9	2.6	8.3	10.1
France	3.3	3.5	6.7	8.1
Germany	3.3	3.5	9.4	10.8

The 2000 figures come from the *Compendium of Health Statistics*: Office of Health Economics 2006; the 2008 figures come from the WHO wesbite.

make the long term commitment to being a partner. Many young doctors didn't want to commit themselves and their families to a long career in a relatively deprived neighbourhood. They were happy to work there for a period but in the long term many aspired to move to wealthier areas with better facilities and good schools for their children.

The established GPs and the profession put up many barriers to increasing the number of salaried GPs. They argued – just as they had in 1948 at the time of the founding of the NHS – that it was important that GPs remained independent practitioners. GPs, they insisted, should not be salaried and allow their professional judgment to be clouded by allegiance to the State or any other employer. Many young GPs, an increasing number of whom were women who wanted a different lifestyle from their predecessors, disagreed. They wanted part time work, the ability to move jobs and freedom from the burden of running a practice.

We had little success at the time but by 2011 all this had changed: 30% of London GPs are salaried and work for other GPs, although not for the State. It suits many of them very well, although some others who want a partnership find it very difficult to get one.

The story suggests both that financial incentives work and reinforces the point that local service leaders can make role changes far more easily than distant managers or governments.

Pay, terms and conditions

The NHS Plan also presaged a very ambitious *pay modernisation* agenda which was designed to simplify the complex arrangements that had grown up since the NHS was founded to link both pay and promotion to enhanced skills and, to some extent, to performance. It would include a job evaluation system and therefore also help deal with equal pay claims which were becoming an issue nationally.

The Department set aside money to implement these changes but also planned for an improvement in value for money as a result of them. In other words the changes would cost more, but they provided some tools which managers could use to make sure that staff worked more efficiently and more productively.

There is an important political background to understand here. Political parties develop their policies in opposition partly through extensive contact with the various interested parties. As a result the Labour Party came into Government with commitments to honour, a history of tension with doctors and close linkages with the trades unions which represented most other staff. These influences helped shape the human resources agenda over the next few years. Ministers had in effect a political mandate to increase staffing levels, tackle doctors' private practice and improve terms and conditions and development opportunities for other staff. There was therefore a political element to everything that was done.

The programme for all staff other than doctors, dentists and senior managers was called "Agenda for Change"[9] and had three elements: harmonised terms and conditions and a single pay spine; a job evaluation scheme; and a competency based staff development framework. It was a massive undertaking to bring together the separate arrangements that covered 54 professions as well as technical, administrative, maintenance and other staff onto a single pay spine and deal with the large numbers of special allowances of various kinds that had grown up over the years.

Remarkably, once agreement was reached, all 1.1 million NHS staff were covered in two years from 2004. This as the National Audit Office (NAO) wrote *"gives the NHS a single and transparent system for employing staff and simplifies significantly the administration of pay within the NHS."*[10]

The NAO questioned at the time whether other benefits including enhanced value for money had been achieved. A later NAO report on hospital productivity in December 2010 did, however, note that labour productivity for the staff groups covered by Agenda for Change increased by 2.3% per annum after implementation between 2005 and 2008, although it said that the precise cause for this couldn't be determined.[11]

The NAO also found it difficult to assess the additional cost of Agenda for Change and suggested that it led to *"a difference in the total pay bill of between minus 0.8 per cent (£239 million) and plus 0.6 per cent (£166 million). The variation is small compared with the actual pay bill figure for 2007-08 of £28,182 million."*[12]

Overall, the NAO reports, my own experience and that of others I have tested it with, lead to the conclusion that whilst we created a much improved framework and controlled costs well, it had taken an enormous amount of effort and difficulty and we had not yet realised the anticipated benefits of the scheme.

The Consultant contract was predictably difficult to negotiate. It had remained largely unchanged from 1948; although since 1991 the Department had been trying to ensure that Consultants were better managed. In 1995 the Audit Commission highlighted concerns about doctors' commitment to the NHS and the failure of most Trusts to manage them effectively.[13] Others expressed similar concerns. For their part the BMA wrote to the Government in 1997 requesting a new contract to address concerns about long hours and pay.

Against this background the negotiation was designed to introduce a stronger contractual framework and to reward the consultants who contributed most to the NHS. Once again there was money set aside to achieve these ends.

There were a number of confounding issues which affected Consultant morale and were to leave a bitter legacy. The Secretary of State, Alan Milburn, made it clear that he wanted to tackle the issue of private practice which since 1948 had bedeviled the NHS. Many Consultants resented this and the idea that they needed to have detailed job plans to account for all their activities. It didn't fit with how they saw themselves as independent professionals. In the same time period the Bristol Royal Infirmary, the Royal Liverpool Children's Hospital and Shipman Inquiries were also damaging the morale and reputation of the profession.

I knew from personal experience as Chief Executive of the Heatherwood and Wexham Park Hospitals NHS Trust before I moved to Oxford that private practice was an issue in some parts of the country and some specialties. Surgeons could earn upwards of £½ million a year from private practice at the time in and around London, on top of an NHS salary of around £75,000. They had access to this private practice because they had their NHS contracts. It is odd that as an employer the NHS allows its most senior people to work freelance or for other employers, sometimes in direct competition with the NHS.

We had to work hard at Heatherwood and Wexham to find ways to manage Consultant's private practice activities so that they didn't interfere with the NHS work and were largely successful. There were hidden influences, however. A very senior doctor told me recently that you had to understand patterns of private practice in London to understand service planning and opposition to some of the hospital reconfigurations.

His point was that a surgeon who drew his private practice from a particular area was certain to resist anything that diminished the role of the NHS hospital there. If he and his NHS practice were transferred to another larger hospital it would put him in competition there for private patients with other surgeons. Similarly I have come across cases where doctors have not wanted to see additional Consultants appointed locally because they would have to share the private practice.

This influence is largely unnoticed. However, the new contract brought greater transparency with a mandatory Code of Contract on Private Practice which requires, inter alia, an annual declaration of when and where each consultant conducts private practice.

These cases are the exception. Most Consultants, particularly away from London, do very little if any private practice. All of them resented the implication that the whole profession was implicated in possible abuse or conflicts of interest. Private practice, however, was something of a totem for the Government. Opposition to private practice had deep historical roots in the Labour Party and a great deal of effort went into thinking up increasingly complex ways of managing it tightly – with, for example, a proposal that Consultants had to do so many hours overtime for the NHS before they could work in the private sector.

The issue influenced the whole tenor of the negotiations and the shape of the contract. It also, after the initial euphoria associated with the NHS Plan died away, helped establish a largely negative relationship between doctors and the Government. This was reinforced as the new policies about patient choice and private sector competition were introduced.

Eventually the new contract was agreed. Consultants had tighter job plans and were more accountable and private practice was more controlled if not eliminated from the NHS. For their part many Consultants had their full contribution to the NHS recognised for the first time and saw their pay rise or their workload reduce. The NAO concluded that "*The contract has delivered some benefits in management of consultant time, prevention of an increase in private practice, securing extra work at plain time and increasing participation. The contract has the capacity to provide some new levers for further enhancing management control (for example, on pay progression) although these have yet to be fully utilised.*"[14] Consultant productivity had been falling for years and the NAO report on hospital productivity showed some improvement, in that the rate of fall reduced after the contract was implemented.[15]

We had budgeted an additional £565 million for implementing the contract but in practice had an estimated overspend of £150 million which was added to NHS budgets in 2005.

Once again the contract had been implemented, some progress had been made and there was a good platform in place for the future. However, the full range of benefits hadn't been achieved and the whole process had been disruptive.

The negotiations with the GPs were rather different because they were concerned with a service contract not an employment one. Here the aim was to make primary care more accessible, offer patients more choice, move more services from secondary to primary care and make primary care an attractive career option at a time when morale was low and recruitment difficult. Once again there was more money on the table. This time the NHS Confederation – the employers' organisation – took the lead in negotiation.

Primary care was critical to the success of the reforms and our proposals were designed to strengthen it and make it more flexible. The contract structure was innovative. It moved from paying individual GPs on the basis of the size of their patient list together with fees for extra services to paying the practice, not the GP, and offering financial incentives for delivering measurable levels of quality and enhanced services. For the first time quality was part of the deal and the evidence based measures chosen – such as monitoring people with cardiac problems or diabetes – were as much concerned with the prevention and management of diseases as with treatment. These were all very good initiatives in principle.

Despite these very considerable advantages – and the NAO saw there being some progress in 11 of the 13 results areas identified in the business plan – there were two big problems.[16] Practices no longer had to manage their "out of hours" services and, even though many already employed locums to do so, the resulting services were perceived to be much worse by the public. The second problem was that the costs of implementation were much higher than intended – by about £816 million in 2005–2006. This was mainly due to setting too low a baseline for the quality measures and assuming that most practices would not achieve as high a level in the first years as they did. A large number of GPs got an unexpected bonus as a result, amounting to an estimated 58% average increase spread over three years.[17]

The "out of hours" and overpayments have been factored into later deals with the GPs and some progress has been made in restoring the position on both. However, other improvement aims were achieved: there is now no problem in recruiting GPs and a strengthened primary care system is in a much better position to take on extra responsibilities in commissioning and elsewhere.

What went wrong?

Progress was made in all these three areas and new and better arrangements were in place at the end of this period. These were massive changes in the largest workforce in Europe. However, the full planned benefits were not realised and implementation caused problems and affected morale. There were three principal reasons for this.

Firstly, we were trying to do a great deal at the same time. These changes were introduced simultaneously with far-reaching service changes, organisational changes and an NHS wide focus on delivering the highest priority clinical and service targets. It is too simple, however, to say that the NHS was overloaded. There is a choice here. Changes were needed and could be planned sequentially and take a very long time indeed – with the potential for missing out on synergies – or everything can be done at the same time with the potential for the sort of problems we saw.

The second reason was a partial disconnect between the people at the centre who negotiated the deals and those locally who had to implement them. This is a potential problem in any organisation but particularly so in one like the NHS where there are disparate centres of power and authority. Even though there were clinical and managerial reference groups involved in the national process, local NHS leaders often felt that they were having unwelcome changes imposed upon them.

The familiar two part approach of performance management and improvement was used in this area and many hours were spent in negotiation between the Delivery Directorate and local NHS organisations over the pace and detail of implementation. However, by this time we were also trying to decentralise and were beginning to lose some of the consistency and grip which went with central control.

The third reason was that the government had too many conflicting roles to play – employer, regulator, payer, fund raiser – and, in the specific case of Labour, champion of the worker and the NHS. It is a familiar problem in other countries where Government is the main driver of health improvement and provider of healthcare and tries to perform too many roles simultaneously. The Government also became very closely associated with the changes thereby effectively politicising many aspects. Moreover, it had political goals and a political timetable to achieve which limited the freedom of manoeuvre of its negotiators.

The HR Director for the NHS who had led most of the changes, Andrew Foster, reflects now that "*Whilst not perfect and implemented with much difficulty it was a major achievement to replace Whitley and the old consultant contract. The new systems created new levers to improve productivity and services in the future – and Trust Chief Executives are increasingly using them now when money is so tight*".

Andrew is now a Trust Chief Executive.

Underlying all these issues is a wide problem of motivation which I will return to in Chapter 9. Making changes in pay and terms and conditions is very difficult, and can de-motivate even when pay increases.

Global connections

At the beginning of this period the NHS was employing increasing numbers of migrant health workers who had trained in Africa and Asia. At its peak in 2002 2,114 South African nurses joined the Nursing and Midwifery Council register in the UK and became eligible to work in the NHS. They were the latest in a long tradition of people, mainly from Commonwealth countries, who had come to work or train in the NHS and who, particularly in the early years, had kept the NHS going. We owe them and their countries a great debt of gratitude.

Since 1997, however, the Government had increased nurse and medical training substantially – with the annual UK intake of medical students going up from 3,000 in 1997 to over 8,000 in 2009 – so as to reach self-sufficiency. Over the same period it introduced ethical recruitment policies to limit entry to people from countries like the Philippines where it had agreements on migration. By 2006 the NHS had effectively become self-sufficient and closed its doors to migrants – with only 37 nurses coming from South Africa in 2007.[18]

Many migrants, particularly doctors from India and other parts of South Asia actually came to the UK primarily for training and many subsequently went home. They wanted to learn from us and acquire our skills and knowledge. Today there is a great deal of scope for the UK to learn from low and middle income countries about many things, including job re-design. In Mozambique, for example, *tecnicos di cirurgia* – often nurses with additional training – do most of the caesareans and, according to long term studies, do them with as few complications as doctors and at much less cost.[19]

These arrangements can't be translated simply to the UK anymore than our practices can be simply transplanted to Mozambique. However, they should make us think – although I imagine it would make the Medical Director I quoted on the first page of this chapter who thought it was illegal for nurses to order X rays absolutely apoplectic to contemplate nurses undertaking caesareans.

Conclusions and key points

1. Restructuring of the workforce and re-design of jobs is essential to deal with changed circumstances and manage costs. Incentives can help but local leaders – in particular doctors – can make significant changes where external managers cannot. The GPs in particular led a great deal of change.

2. All the HR policies were linked to the *skills escalator* whereby an individual could progress up the organisation gaining experience, skills and reward on the way; whilst roles could be passed down the organisation as new systems and technology allowed and appropriate systems were put in place.

3. There were many problems recruiting staff at the beginning of the period but improved pay and terms of conditions as well as higher levels of education and training meant that target levels of increases in staffing were exceeded.

4. Wider policy issue such as the European Working Times Directive and changes in taxation affect health policy and costs.

5. The major programmes for changing pay and terms and conditions created streamlined and more flexible arrangements, but many benefits were not realised in the short term – and, in the GPs contract, led to large cost over runs.

6. The difficulties in implementation were largely due to: doing many things at the same time; a disconnect between the people negotiating and those implementing which was reinforced by increasing decentralisation; and Government playing too many roles from funder to negotiator and NHS champion. Some issues also became very politicised. Managers need to choose whether to make changes sequentially or concurrently – either way there will be problems that need to be managed.

7. Underlying all these issues is a wider problem of motivation. Making changes in pay and terms and conditions is very difficult, and can de-motivate even when pay increases.

References

1. Department of Health (2002) *HR in the NHS Plan;* July, para 4.8, p 15.
2. Jarman B, Gault S, Alves B, Hider A, Dolan S, Cook A, Hurwitz B, Lezzoni LI (1999) Explaining differences in English hospital death rates using routinely collected data. *BMJ* **318**: 1515.

3. Starfield B, Shi L, Grover A, Mackino J (2005) The effects of specialist supply on populations' health: assessing the evidence. *Health Aff (Millwood)* March 2005.
4. Williams J, Dural D, Cheung WY *et al.* (2009) Effectiveness of nurse delivered endoscopy: findings from randomised mulli-institution nurse endoscopy trial (MINUET). *BMJ* **338**: 231.
5. *NHS Staffing Overview 2009*: NHS Information Centre. 25 March 2010.
6. Ibid.
7. Ibid.
8. Ibid.
9. Department of Health (1999) *Agenda for change: Modernising the NHS pay system*; Feb.
10. National Audit Office (2009) *NHS Pay Modernisation in England: Agenda for Change*; TSO 27, Jan, para 24, p 8.
11. National Audit Office (2010) *Management of NHS Hospital Productivity*; 17 Dec, figure 6 p 16.
12. Ibid. para 2.18, p18.
13. The Audit Commission (1995) *The Doctors' Tale: the Work of Hospital Doctors in England and Wales*.
14. National Audit Office (2007) *Pay Modernisation: A new contract for Consultants in England*: 19 April, para 26, p 6.
15. National Audit Office (2010) *Management of NHS Hospital Productivity*; 17th Dec, figure 6, p 16.
16. National Audit Office (2008) *NHS Pay Modernisation: New contracts for general practice services in England.* 28 Feb.
17. Ibid. para 17, p 4.
18. Midwifery and Nursing Council: statistical analysis of the register.
19. Kruk ME, Pereira C, Vaz F, Bergstrom S, Gales S (2007) Economic evaluation of surgically trained assistant medical officers in performing major obstetric surgery in Mozambique. *Br J Obstet Gynaecol* **114**: 1253–60.

Chapter 7

Knowledge, science and technology

By 2006 we had the largest digital imaging network in the world and the ability to pass CT scans and other images around the country. It meant, for example, that anyone who had a head injury at night could have a scan taken at their local hospital which could be transmitted to the home of whichever specialist radiological Consultant was on duty that night in the region. Previously a local radiologist would have read the scan and then, if they needed to, discussed it over the phone with whoever they could contact. The best opinion was now a click away.

Meanwhile, the digital imaging systems being installed in every acute hospital meant that there would be no more lost images and clinicians could have them available to them wherever they needed them in the clinic or the ward. Previously up to 10% of X rays had to be repeated because the films were lost. Quality, decision making and costs were all improved by the new systems.

This is excellent, but these gains could be taken much further. Some parts of the country haven't taken out all the costs they might; preferring, for example, to see the specialist rota as an add-on rather than a substitute for their own services. Similar systems could be put in place for pathology so that histological images could be sent to and viewed at a specialist centre. Do we still need 27 laboratories in London? More radically, images could be sent to India or elsewhere for interpretation.

The electronic prescription system, which was also installed by this date, meant that anyone who needed repeat prescriptions, as many middle aged and elderly people do, could have their re-fills sent to their home, cutting out the tedious trips to the pharmacy. Yet five years later this is still rarely available to patients and few know it is an option; perhaps because it would challenge the viability of local pharmacies, many of which are run by GP practices.

There may be reasons why some of these improvements wouldn't work in specific cases but it is unlikely to be true everywhere. These examples of advances in technology reinforce the points made in the last chapter about the importance of workforce re-structuring and job re-design. They also remind us of the likely sources of resistance – the individuals whose skills are no longer needed and will require re-training or lose their jobs; the hospitals or practices that will lose revenue as services move; and the professions which fear a loss of power as their authority diminishes. All these concerns will be wrapped up in the old battle cry – *"we must keep our local service"* – even if the alternative is better quality and less cost.

The application of knowledge, evidence and technology

This chapter is about knowledge, evidence, technology and their application. They were fundamental to everything that was done in implementing the NHS Plan: whether we were developing the National Services Frameworks for Mental Health or Diabetes; identifying and spreading best practice through the Modernisation Agency; applying the most up to date technology for IT; or building the clinical knowledge base through research and development (R and D).

Central to my role as Chief Executive was trying to understand how best to apply that knowledge – global best practice wherever possible – to the vast organisation of the NHS with its myriad opportunities and problems.

In IT, with which we start this chapter, we had recruited Richard Granger with world class experience in major public sector IT applications to lead implementation. Elsewhere other great leaders like Andrew Dillon and Mike Rawlins at NICE, Muir Gray in knowledge management and Sally Davies in R and D worked to make knowledge available in the NHS.

This chapter provides a brief insight into their work: moving from IT to design and building, on to evidence and knowledge management and concluding with R and D. Not everything can be covered here but my aim is to illustrate some of the things done in each area, identify lessons and demonstrate how important knowledge, science and technology were as the fourth area of reform.

The National Programme for IT

The National Programme for IT (NPfIT), later *Connecting for Health*, was created in 2002 at a time when we were beginning to understand what a transformative impact IT could have in healthcare.

It was the biggest civil IT programme in the world, only the US military was bigger, and had many components. At its heart were the two goals of enabling the NHS to connect all its parts successfully and supporting local NHS organisations to acquire and use the best applications for their purposes. Both facilitate the appropriate use of knowledge and help improve quality and costs.

There were no ready made solutions on the market; the NHS was at the forefront and pioneering new solutions once again. I well remember Richard Granger soon after his appointment in late 2002 telling suppliers with his customary vigour that the industry would have to re-shape itself to meet our needs. There were, he said, some organisations with the capability to support the programme but without the capacity to do so at scale and some large organisations with the reach but not the capability. They needed to get their act together if they wanted any of his budget.

It was an approach that stood him and us in good stead throughout the procurement process. Richard mobilised staff and resources quickly and was able to let all the main contracts within the year from February 2003 and do so with an independently estimated cost saving of £4.5 billion and with tough performance measures in place.[1] It was a revelation for Government and a shock to the industry.

Richard's approach subsequently changed Government policy on procurement and outsourcing – never again could Government be seen as an easy touch. Some of the private sector organisations, which were very keen to have as much as possible of these lucrative contracts sought to lobby ministers and Number 10, complaining of his approach and saying he was driving too hard a bargain.

Chief Executives of the big IT companies would go and see ministers and tell them just how much they wanted to support the Government's programme but that they had opportunities elsewhere and might have to move some part of their UK operations overseas. Ministers held their nerve; the IT companies blinked … and signed the contracts.

I was to see the same tactics employed later, however, with some success by the pharmaceutical companies when we were re-negotiating drug prices.

There was another innovative aspect. Many large organisations at the time contracted implementation of their IT programmes to a single company or consortium. Once contracts were signed they were at the mercy of the supplier. In order to avoid this risk NPfIT tendered for Local Service Providers in five areas which covered the whole country. Four companies secured contracts; one won two areas.

In a memorable image Richard told the suppliers that he was operating on the "husky principle". If one husky in a team fails to perform it is cut out of the traces and fed to the others. It was both a threat and an incentive. If one of the contractors failed to perform the others would get more business.

These contracts were very valuable.

There has been a great deal of confusion about the total costs of the Programme in part depending on whether this means only the cost of putting the Programme in place or whether it also includes the cost of running it each year. Moreover the NHS spends a great deal on IT systems that are not part of the Programme and are not covered in its costs.

I have followed here the definitions used by the independent National Audit Office (NAO). In 2006 the NAO report a total anticipated gross cost of £12.4 billion for implementing the Programme, without including running costs or any other NHS spend on IT and without any reduction for savings as a result of the Programme. At that time the Department had already identified savings of £208 million from the programme and anticipated more than £1.1 billion to be saved in running costs over the 10 year period from 2003.[2]

The actual spend has been less than planned due to slow progress with the care records system and to suppliers incurring "delay deductions", which they could earn back if performance improved. At 31 March 2008 spending on the Programme was almost £1.5 billion behind the original profile.[3] Management of the contracts remained appropriately tough. One of the four Local Service Providers had failed and duly been "eaten" by others. As the NAO puts it:

> "NHS Connecting for Health has taken positive action to ensure that contractors are managing their tasks well. It has taken an intrusive but supportive approach to the management of suppliers. Where it has identified problems, NHS Connecting for Health has taken action to address deficiencies in suppliers' performance".[4]

Procurement went very well but progress with implementation was mixed. Some elements have been delivered: the new national network (N3) is in place as is the NHS Directory; the electronic prescription service; "Choose and Book" – the system enabling patients to book admissions and outpatient appointments – and the demographic service. These are all enormous projects in their own right. At the same time there have been a very large number of local deployments of software, 9,600 by April 2006, including new hospital Patient Administration Systems – the core local system – and 30 of the planned imaging systems.[5]

However, there were major problems in the highest profile area: the NHS Care Records Service which would make summaries of patients' records available throughout the NHS. There have been delays, technical problems and, significantly, difficulties in working with local NHS organisations. These problems fatally damaged the image and reputation of the whole Programme. It is the part of the reforms which has attracted the most criticism, and therefore it is important to understand what went wrong.

It is not easy to disentangle the various different causes for these problems. In part they were due to the novelty and complexity of what was being attempted. The main causes, however, seem to have been around design, the centralised approach and changes in the implementation model.

In retrospect it is easy to argue that the design was too rigid. With hindsight two questions stand out: how far was it necessary to standardise hospital system within each of the five clusters and was it essential to have all hospital PAS systems permanently interconnected to the spine in real time? Today, with the whole field having progressed, we might well consider that other perhaps more web-based technical solutions could be better. If we move on a few more years then today's solutions may well look out of date.

This was connected with our centralised approach. When the programme was started the NHS had literally 1,000s of different systems with little communication between them inside organisations, let alone between them. We consciously took the decision to centralise and standardise so as to get maximum benefit from the ability to link and share both information and the implementation process. We reasoned, amongst other things, that the NHS should not go through the same learning process time and time again but, working together, learn and implement at the same time.

The excellence and the speed of procurement which was such an advantage also had a downside. There was relatively little time for consultation which might both have achieved greater buy in and improved the design. Adaptations were made as implementation progressed but were inevitably more difficult to put in place.

We had initially planned to use our well developed model for implementation of the Modernisation Agency and clinical leaders working to identify and spread good practice on the one hand and the Delivery Directorate holding organisations to account for performance on the other. There were, however, two difficulties.

Firstly, whilst we appointed clinicians nationally and regionally to help steer the whole process as national directors and advisers, there was very little clinical consensus about what needed to be done. As a result the clinical leaders' expertise was much more open to challenge than it was for the Czars in cancer and emergency care. Many doctors around the country had their own views about and, sometimes, extensive experience in IT and clinical systems. This lack of clinical agreement was very problematic and led to complaints that doctors weren't fully involved.

Secondly, these implementation plans were damaged by our own decentralisation policies which were coming into affect at the same time. Foundation Trusts were just being established which, because of their legal status, could opt out of most, but not all, of the national programme if they chose. As part of the same process of devolving power we broke up and decentralised the Modernisation Agency.

These two changes reduced our leverage. Implementing major new systems in a managed organisation with clear accountabilities was one thing, doing so in a system where we were also telling organisations that we wanted them to be more independent was quite another. In the event we had to rely much more on persuasion and local leadership than on systematic project management. It was a bumpy ride.

Politics was another confounding factor. The Government set out its ambitions at the start and raised expectations very high. This left them and the programme open to political attack, which duly came – with the whole programme and Richard Granger in particular victims of some startling aggressive tactics.

The final factor was the weight of other priorities and activities that the NHS was dealing with simultaneously. Here as elsewhere I had Chief Executives asking me: "*What are the most important priorities – waiting lists, cancer, the consultant contract, IT, my new hospital, the budget or patient choice? How do you want me to focus my limited management time? Which will I get sacked for if I don't deliver?*"

This account raises the same policy choices as we saw with the staff contracts: would it have been better to do all the major reforms in sequence, even though this would be enormously lengthy and might lose synergy, or was it better to implement them at the same time, risking disruption and failing to realise all the benefits on time? Was it right to raise the profile and thereby get a good degree of energy and urgency behind the programme or would it have been better to be slower and more low key?

This short account describes a continuing programme which has already delivered a whole series of gains for the NHS – who today would want to be without digital imaging, the secure messaging service or the patient demography index? The procurement process set a new standard for the public sector, the programme is under spent and the NHS has powerful contracts to keep suppliers up to the mark. In practice implementation has become more localised and some of the rigidities have been removed.

Nevertheless the public perception is of a programme that has not delivered on the central goal of integrated patient record available across the NHS.

It may be that once the immediate noise and controversy has dissipated, as with the staff contracts, that the programme will be seen to have been useful in creating a platform for further improvement. The NHS will undoubtedly need to use its IT systems to secure some of the more radical improvements in services and costs that I described at the beginning of the chapter.

There are some unresolved issues such as confidentiality of patient information. There is more scope for damaging breaches of confidentiality with electronic records where an accidental key stroke could send a record anywhere around the system. Safeguards to reduce the chances of this happening were installed; but there is still a great deal of public debate to be had on this issue. Greater understanding is needed of how people value having an electronic record that just might possibly help save their life as against the risk of a breach of confidentiality.

As with workforce restructuring, GPs have progressed quite quickly in this field. The Quality Management and Analysis System – the programme designed to measure GP performance and thereby authorise their increased income as a result of their new contract – was perhaps not surprisingly implemented very quickly. There was no clinical opposition! Meanwhile GPs, who run their practices as their own small businesses, have implemented effective internal IT systems for doing so. Financial incentives and independence are very powerful motivators.

This is an important pointer for the future but also raises questions. Bottom up change is clearly very important, but how much top down leadership is also needed? These GP systems were much simpler that other parts of the National Programme. Could GPs, for example, implement an NHS wide system like the secure network? Would they ensure that full advantage would be taken of a system like the prescribing one where the benefits to the whole NHS might come in part at their own expense? I will return to the question of implementing large scale change in looking to the future in Chapter 12.

Design and building

The design of buildings is also fundamentally important in improving quality and costs. It too requires the knowledge and understanding of what is most effective in practice and the application of appropriate technologies.

My Friday visits to different parts of the NHS gave me a vivid picture of the problems on the NHS estate at the end of the 90s. I saw mental health wards where people lived for long periods in old, cramped, unfit accommodation with little privacy and few facilities. These were not the long stay asylums of old, hidden from public view, but facilities used for acute admissions of people who were despairing or psychotic and needed comfort and rehabilitation and the space and time for recovery. Psychiatrists and nurses told me how important the environment could be as an aid to healing. I could see for myself how the design and architecture lowered the spirits and shrank the world.

I recall one A and E Department in west London, now thankfully gone, which was separated by open walkways from the wards and departments and where patients were wheeled on trolleys through the open air or taken on an old electric ambulance to the wards. I knew another hospital in north London, by no means unique, where dying patients were nursed in narrow old fashioned wards where their relatives found themselves constantly in the way of busy members of staff.

There were, of course, some very good facilities but the overwhelming sense of the NHS estate at that time was of unplanned sites where each generation's new development – sometimes solidly built and sometimes temporary buildings – had been squeezed in wherever they would fit around and between, underneath and above existing facilities. Too often the whole site had been neglected with maintenance budgets cut in favour of direct patient care. Primary care in inner cities was as bad with surgeries in terraced houses or pre-fabs with no room for practice nurses or new equipment and utterly unsuited to aspirations for a world class service.

The NHS Plan set out wide ranging plans to build new hospitals and surgeries, promising capital investment of at least £7 billion on at least 100 new hospital projects and 3,000 refurbishments in primary care and thereby reducing the backlog maintenance costs estimated at £3 billion by 25%.[6]

All of this was delivered and more.

The rejuvenation of the NHS estate

The NHS Plan initiated an extraordinary rejuvenation of NHS estates: redundant sites and buildings were sold off – old mental hospitals making surprisingly good apartments – and a new generation of hospitals appeared, accompanied by diagnostic and treatment centres (DTCs), GP practices, primary and community care facilities, walk-in centres and, of course, better and more humane mental health and secure facilities.

As this list shows, there were also serious efforts to diversify the estate and support the new services described in Chapter 4 by creating facilities that would enable us to bring together primary, community and social care; make services more accessible to patients and bring more doctors into the sorts of multi-partner practices we believed were generally preferable. The estate began to support the move from a hospital and doctor centric service to a more community based one where services were delivered by a range of staff and involved the patients themselves.

By 2000 the Central Middlesex Ambulatory Care and Diagnostic Centre (ACAD) – designed to focus on ambulatory, not inpatient care – had already replaced a large part of an older hospital built on the traditional model of wards and departments. In the ACAD everything was brought together around the diagnostic and therapeutic processes with radiology, pathology and physiotherapy services available where they were needed, not separate and distant. It was a design model for the future.

There were, as ever, complicating factors. The new model diminished the role of the traditional District General Hospital – a local hospital providing a comprehensive range of acute services – and often led reformers who wanted to move services away from such hospitals into conflict with local people anxious to defend the hospital they knew and loved.

Sometimes as at the Central Middlesex, the local Trust was able to take the public with them when they got rid of inpatient beds and replaced them with other facilities. More often there was conflict with people whose interests were tied up in the existing hospital when local services were "threatened": sometimes the patterns of doctors' private practice were involved, often the unions were but the local MP and other politicians were always fully engaged. It takes a brave MP to support closure of the A and E Department or inpatient beds in his or her constituency. Changing service models is difficult in any country and the issue still needs to be resolved in the NHS today. When Lord Darzi brought forward his proposals in 2007 to develop new local services across London it provoked just these sorts of problems. Such plans were put on hold by the Coalition Government.[7] They are however going to have to face up to it sooner rather than later.

The other problem was the familiar one that the Government set a target for more inpatient beds in the NHS Plan in what appeared to be a response to public and media pressure. This was rather like the targets on the workforce. More staff were needed in very specific areas, however the targets drove increases everywhere. More intermediate and low-tech beds were needed in the community but the targets led to higher than necessary numbers in some new hospital developments. This brought short term gains in the media but created longer term problems. Arguably, too many acute beds were developed in London and not enough was done to increase intermediate and longer term accommodation for older people.

These developments have been partially funded by the increase in NHS capital but about two thirds had some element of private finance involved. In 1997 there was little expertise in the public or private sectors about how to make this work and considerable time and effort was spent in learning how to create the right relationships as well as the right contracts; how to streamline lengthy processes and, crucially, how to ensure that high quality design was involved in creating buildings fit for the future.

The NHS had been starved of capital funding for years, the private sector wanted the work and the politicians wanted results. We were all in a hurry. It was in some ways a bad combination: and some of the early projects were not fully thought through and did not reflect our aspirations for quality and new designs. Later, however, the necessary expertise was developed on all sides and some excellent buildings were built. Importantly, this was not limited to hospitals but in creating NHS Local Improvement Finance Trusts (NHS Lift), the Department was able to bring together local NHS organisations with local businesses and investors to fund "bundles" of small primary and community developments. This has been very successful in many areas.

The implications of using private finance for public development are discussed in the next chapter in the context of the wider finances of the NHS. The central point here is that it was a major contributor to the resuscitation of the NHS estate. Today we can go to almost any major NHS site and see some and perhaps many buildings we can be proud of. They are symbols of and contributors to high quality care. It was very different in 1999.

Few Chief Executives in the NHS are very conversant with design and estates issues and, unless they had a major project underway, leave much of the detail to their experts. In the future, however, I believe that these issues need to rise up the agenda. There is plenty of evidence both about how design enhances patient care and about how it reduces costs and improves the operation of organisations and services.[8] Additionally, environmental and sustainability issues are now coming much more to the fore with NHS organisations expected to play their part in reducing carbon usage and enhancing the environment.[9]

Knowledge and evidence

Over the last two decades and more the UK has played a leading role in making evidence available for clinicians and patients. In 1993 Sir Muir Gray supported Sir Iain Chalmers in the establishment of the Cochrane Collaboration as "*an international network of people helping healthcare providers, policy makers, patients,* *their advocates and carers, make well-informed decisions about human health care by preparing, updating and promoting the accessibility of **Cochrane Reviews**".*[10]

These reviews analyse all the available research on a specific question and assess what conclusions can be drawn. Over 4,500 reviews have so far been published on line in the Cochrane Library.

This remarkable organisation has spread around the world and affected health policy profoundly. In 2011 it was accepted as a Non-Governmental Organization in Official Relations with the WHO thus establishing a partnership which will strengthen its influence still further.

There are many linkages with today's efforts to improve health and healthcare. Muir Gray, with his enormous enthusiasm and energy, has often been part of them. I recall how when I arrived as Chief Executive in the Oxford Radcliffe in 1993 he led me from my office to the onsite bookshop and bought me David Sackett's latest book on evidence based decision making.[11] He was determined that managers as well as clinicians should understand the importance of evidence and knowledge.

Muir has gone on to develop other ways of promoting knowledge and evidence such as the creation of the NHS Electronic Library of Health. He subsequently became the first Knowledge Director of the NHS with responsibility for findings ways to strengthen the knowledge base and its use throughout the organisation.

More recently he has taken a new role in promoting the way health systems can incorporate knowledge most effectively into their processes and operations and in which citizen access to knowledge can revolutionise services. Muir argues that the proper application of what is already known would have a greater impact than any new technology likely to be invented in the next decade, and that clean clear knowledge would be as important in the 21st century as clean clear water had been in the 19th.[12]

NICE: the appraisal of therapies and access to evidence

In the late 90s the new Government set out to strengthen quality in the NHS and create better evidence for the use of therapies and better guidance for clinicians. In 1999 the National Institute for Health and Clinical Excellence (NICE) was established to *"ensure everyone has equal access to medical treatments and high quality care from the NHS - regardless of where they live in England and Wales".*[13]

NICE started out with a clear remit to focus on "technology appraisals" – appraising medicines, treatments and technologies; but over the years has done increasingly more to make recommendations on how to care for people with specific diseases and conditions. In 2005 its responsibilities were widened beyond the clinical to include issuing guidance on how to improve peoples' health and prevent illness and death.

NICE has been remarkably successful over the years and now has a range of programmes including NHS Evidence – a Google style device for identifying evidence and best practice that grew out of the Electronic Library; the development of quality standards for the NHS; and overseeing the development of the quality and outcome indicators used in the new GP contract. By June 2010 it had undertaken 217 technology appraisals with 125 underway and issued 705 pieces of guidance with 240 underway. It is the largest issuer of clinical guidelines in the world.

In the words of the Chief Executive, Sir Andrew Dillon, *"We try to use whatever opportunity we helpfully can to make evidence available to everyone – the public and clinicians alike"*.

NICE has been seen as highly controversial, particularly regarding its new drug appraisals. A lot of this is based on misunderstandings and, to some extent, what appears to be deliberate misinformation about its role. In these appraisals NICE reviews all the evidence about a therapy, considers what its advisory groups say, and looks at its effectiveness and cost effectiveness. It is thus able to comment on comparative effectiveness and therefore, for example, on whether a new product on the market is actually any better than existing ones. This distinguishes NICE from the formal regulatory bodies such as the Food and Drugs Administration (FDA) in the US, which only consider safety and efficacy and do not make comparisons. Their task is to licence not to compare and advise.

One common misunderstanding is that NICE guidance prevents the NHS from using certain therapies. In fact the only mandatory aspect of NICE is that an NHS organisation must pay for any treatment it recommends if clinicians locally choose to prescribe it. Clinicians can prescribe anything else that is legal and NHS organisations can pay for them if they choose. Individuals and private health schemes can pay for what they want. NICE's actual power is to insist that certain therapies are paid for by the NHS not to stop others being prescribed or paid for. The effect of its guidance, however, is rather different.

In practice many organisations both NHS and private do treat NICE guidance as the standard to adhere to and as defining what can be provided – on the grounds of what the evidence shows as well as for financial considerations. This was one of the main reasons why pharmaceutical organisations lobbied so strongly against NICE in my time: they feared that it set an evidence based standard that people in other countries would also regard as the norm.

NICE is also unique in appraising therapies in terms of cost utility. It calculates the cost of using the therapy to achieve an additional year of quality life for an individual – or a "Quality Adjusted Life Year" (QUALY). It uses a benchmark figure of £30,000 per QUALY, although it can and does on occasion agree to support the use of interventions at a higher figure.

It is worth noting that NICE does not make recommendations on costs and QUALYS in areas such as Intensive Care or Special Care Babies Units where the "rule of rescue" applies – whereby clinicians do whatever they can to rescue the patient in front of them at whatever cost. Its role is in looking at therapies where clinicians and patients have a choice of therapy and discretion as to whether to use it.

Controversy about NICE focuses on the few occasions a year when it makes an unpopular recommendation on a high profile therapy – often in cases where drugs seem to make a difference for a short term but have little impact on mortality. These are very difficult to address and people have their own views. I have argued that in cases like this where the numbers of people affected are very small the NHS should choose to fund them out of compassion rather than on the evidence and that on a wider basis, where the evidence is poor, that patients should be able to pay for the drug alongside their NHS treatment.[14,15] Neither of these arguments challenges the importance of having the evidence identified and analysed by NICE.

Andrew Dillon, who like his Chairman Sir Michael Rawlins has been in post since its foundation, believes that NICE's success rests on five things. It is independent from Government which can ask it to look at certain therapies or areas but has never challenged its findings. It has close relationships with patient advocates, involving members of patients' organisations in its advisory groups as well as engaging them in consultation. It has a clear set of methods and processes. It operates completely transparently. It has a close relationship with the NHS because so many of the members of its advisory group work in or with the NHS or are its patients. This gives it a close understanding of the clinical context and prevents it from being a distant academic expert out of touch with reality.

There have been critics of some of its processes: that they are too slow, that not all therapies are covered, not all sources of expertise drawn on and its terminology can be difficult for patients to understand.[16] NICE has responded and continues to develop its role.[17] However, it is notable that when the Coalition Government recently seemed to suggest that its role should be diminished, organisations from across the spectrum of healthcare and academia rose to its defence. There is a place for an independent body to weigh the evidence and bring sometimes unpalatable truths into view.

For my part as Chief Executive NICE served very well to separate Ministers from decision making on these matters; which otherwise, as had happened in the past, might have degenerated into straight politics. It also seemed to me at the time no more than common sense to have a good means of assessing whether the major components in the £8 billion we spent on drugs in 2005 were effective and worth the money.

Promoting innovation

The promotion of innovation and the introduction of new technologies into the NHS began to become higher profile issues during the NHS Plan period. Some of the problems were organisational and systemic. The NHS was a largely de-centralised organisation which meant that innovation had to proceed mainly unit by unit. Moreover, changes in clinical practice had to proceed clinician by clinician as each decided whether he or she would use the new therapy or approach. We noted in Chapter 4 how slowly best clinical practice spread unless there was some sort of accelerant like a target or a collaborative process.

There was another dimension to this which involved the healthcare supplies industry from pharmaceuticals to medical devices and consumable products like bandages and sutures. Over the years they had concentrated on selling to individual clinicians and purchasing managers as the key decision makers. Now however, as the emphasis shifted to more managed processes they wanted to be able to get to the general managers and lead clinicians who designed the services and thereby determined which purchases got priority. Purchasing, too, like IT and estates was becoming more integrated into the overall management of the NHS at every level and the industry had to change its approach.

This was a cultural change that was difficult for both sides. There were complaints by industry to Ministers that the NHS wasn't using new technology – or in the case of NICE, as they saw it, slowing down the adoption of innovation. Industry had several problems here: the new managerial culture; decentralisation; and a new NHS assertiveness as a customer which was exemplified by NICE and by Richard Granger's approach to procurement. The big pharmaceuticals companies had the further problem that the development of new drugs is extremely lengthy and expensive and they were being out-competed by new bio-tech companies. Their whole business model was in trouble.

For its part many people in the NHS mistrusted these big industries and could point to many examples of poor practice, withholding of relevant information and manipulation of clinicians through funding their training and other programmes.

Both sides, however, needed to create a new relationship. There were a number of important collaborations over the next few years as industry, Government, the NHS and academia worked through their common issues. In 1999 following a meeting between the Prime Minister and the CEOs of the then three UK based pharmaceutical companies it was agreed to set up the Pharmaceutical Industry Competitiveness Task Force (PICTIF). Its founding purpose was to support the continuing competitiveness of the UK industry which felt that despite a very successful UK record – the UK was 4% of the world pharma market but had more than 10% of the research and had developed 25 of the last 100 best selling drugs – its home market of the NHS didn't value or support it.

PICTIF was successful in building greater trust and understanding and made a series of recommendations about industry engagement in NHS planning, the sharing of information and the development of relationships at local and national level. In 2004 we followed this up with a more informal series of meetings which were chaired by Sir Bill Castell, CEO of GE Healthcare, and me and which involved leading academics. These meetings looked at shared interests and goals with a view to making the most of the assets we had in the UK in our universities, industry and the extraordinary scale and reach of the NHS.

Research and development

There were a further series of reports and actions over the next few years which built up these relationships and are starting to create a health bio-science industry platform which has the capability to serve the UK very well.

The Department's Director General of R and D, Dame Sally Davies now the Chief Medical Officer, has been instrumental both in steering the R and D budget towards greater funding of applied research that is directly relevant to the NHS and in bringing the parties together. I recall her telling me in the late 1990s when we worked together in London that her dream was to see the NHS as a learning laboratory constantly feeding back the results of research into benefits for patients and the public. Her 2006 strategy document for the NHS started to make this a reality by building better links within the NHS – so that research programmes could be networked across the country – and coordinated with the work of the funders.[18]

Sally's thinking was in line with others and in 2006 Sir David Cooksey's report recommended new relationships between the Department's R and D programme, the Medical Research Council and other funding bodies and the establishment by competition of 11 bio-medical research centres for excellence around the country. It also sketched out thoughts about how Pharma and the NHS might cooperate better in drug development to the benefit of both.[19] The Academy of Medical Sciences in 2010 described how to draw the parties closer together to "reap the rewards" for the UK and its patients.[20] The Office for the Strategic Coordination of Health Research, chaired by Sir John Bell, now works to provide the necessary coordination and horizon scanning and help reap the rewards.

There is more to do but there now appears to be a very positive basis for ensuring that the NHS, the UK and the public can benefit from advances in science and technology. The tests will be whether this can survive the recession – which has already brought some industry dis-investments from the UK – and how far these partners can really help make the NHS sustainable. They could play a major role by providing the evidence and offering support and leadership for transferring to the new service and health models from the old.

These partners – the Department, the NHS, academia, research institutes and industry – can also take a wider leadership position as science opens up the opportunities for personalised medicine and for ever more sophisticated understandings of disease and possible treatments.

There are potential downsides to the current explosion in scientific discovery. It could lead to a renewed focus on treatment rather than prevention. It could exclude the poor. It could lead us as patients to be even more dependent on our clinicians and scientists.

The partners and the UK platform they are building could alternatively focus on:

- securing early health not treatment of late disease
- access to all not the few
- promoting science and technologies that help us to be independent, not constantly dependent on drugs and interventions.

The most crucial issue here, however, is the relationship between what is a global public good and what is appropriately private and can be commercialised for profit. This wide ranging partnership may have a role in helping to determine this.

These are all fundamental issues for the future but outside the scope of this book.

Conclusions and key points

1. The National Programme for IT had many successes in improving patient care and costs – from digitised images to the secure NHS network and electronic prescribing – which put England amongst the world leaders in the field. The procurement process was robust and effective, changing Government policy and putting the NHS in a strong position with its suppliers. Costs were well controlled.

2. Problems mainly with the Care Records Service have, however, damaged the reputation of the whole Programme. These were due to design issues, over-centralisation and midstream changes in the implementation programme. These problems were compounded by politics, by difficulties in providing clinical leadership and lack of agreement amongst clinicians and by the range of other priorities facing NHS organisations.

3. The model of implementation used elsewhere, on clinical issues like MRSA and waiting times didn't work here where clinicians had no special knowledge. There are many lessons to learn about managing large scale change involving thousands of people.

4. The NHS estate has been rejuvenated with more than 100 new hospital developments and 3,000 refurbishments in primary care. New buildings and new designs are helping support the more diverse and flexible range of services needed in the future. PFI has been crucial. Here as elsewhere the rush to achieve targets wasted some opportunities for redesign but over time new and better processes have been established.

5. The UK plays a leading role internationally in generating evidence and in knowledge management. NICE has strengthened its role in providing evidence for patients as well as clinicians and policy makers. It is essential to have an independent organisation to identify evidence and knowledge, challenge common assumptions and sometimes reveal unpalatable truths.

6. Introducing innovation in healthcare is difficult for local reasons to do with the structure and culture of the NHS but is also influenced by the wider ways in which clinicians adapt and learn.

7. NHS leaders increasingly need to understand and integrate the contribution that these technical issues – IT, design and knowledge management – play in developing and delivering high quality services.

8. There has been very good progress in R and D in creating a focus on service issues and in developing the NHS as a learning laboratory. The Department, the NHS, academia, research institutes and industry have made progress in coming together to create a common platform for the benefit of patients and the UK.

9. There are policy issues to address about how much science and technology can focus on early health not late disease; provide access to all not just the few; and help create independence rather than dependence – and in doing so create global public goods, not purely private products for commercial exploitation.

References

1. National Audit Office: *Department of Health (2006) The National Programme for IT in the NHS;* 16 June, para d, p 2.
2. National Audit Office (2008) *The National Programme for IT in the NHS: progress since 2006;* 16 May, para 20, p 4.
3. Ibid. para 16, p 4.
4. National Audit Office: Department of Health (2006) *The National Programme for IT in the NHS;* 16 June, para h, p 3.
5. Ibid. para l, p 4.
6. Department of Health: *The NHS Plan – a plan for investment, a plan for reform;* CM 4818-I paras 4.6–4.11, p 44.
7. Department of Health (2007) *Our NHS our future: NHS Next Stage Review:* Oct.
8. Sadler BL, Berry LL, Guenther R, *et al.* (2011) *Fable Hospital 2.0: The Business Case for Building Better Health Care Facilities;* Hastings Centre Report 41, no 1: 13–23.
9. Department of Health (2011) *Route Map for Sustainable Health:* Sustainable Development Unit; Feb.
10. The Cochrane Collaboration website.
11. David L Sackett, R Brian Haynes, Gordon H Guyatt, Peter Tugwell (1991) *Clinical Epidemiology – a basic science for clinical medicine,* 2nd edn; Little, Brown and Co.
12. Pang T, Gray M and Evans T (2006) A 15th grand challenge for global public health. *Lancet* **367**: 284–6.
13. NICE website.
14. Nigel Crisp (2008) Don't let cancer controversy destroy the NHS; *The Times* 24 Sept.
15. Illora Finlay and Nigel Crisp (2008) Drugs for cancer and co-payments. *BMJ* Editorial **337**; 7760 a527 5 July.
16. House of Commons: *Select Committee on Health First Report 2007/08.*
17. House of Commons: *Select Committee on Health First Special Report 2007/08.*
18. Department of Health (2006) *Best research for best health: a new national health research strategy;* 25th Jan.
19. Sir David Cooksey (2006) A review of health research funding; TSO for HM Treasury, Dec.
20. Academy of Medical Sciences (2010) *Reaping the rewards: a vision for UK medical science,* Jan.

Chapter 8

Finance and productivity

As we walked down the corridor we could see that there was an elderly lady standing uncertainly outside the double doors. We asked if we could help her.

"I'm looking for day surgery"

"This is it, you've found it"

"Oh," she said, "I thought this must be for private patients".

It was a revealing and rather sad story. She thought that that the new day surgery unit looked too nice and inviting to be for NHS patients. Her expectations of the NHS were obviously very low. The new furniture, good lighting, clean and pleasant surroundings and neat looking staff had all misled her into thinking she had strayed into the wrong place. We reassured her and she went in to be greeted by a friendly looking receptionist.

It wasn't the only time I came across such a reaction. I was on one of my Friday visits and the Trust Chief Executive with me was doing what they had mostly learned to do by this time and was showing me some of the best services and some of the worst. I wanted to know where the money was going and over the years saw a succession of bright new units and buildings and sometimes whole new hospitals. The NHS was picking itself up off the floor and beginning to look like a world class service.

I also saw some of the worst facilities: blood transfusion and other kidney services being delivered in old mews stables in west London; a GP surgery occupying two unconnected rooms on different floors of a 60s maisonette block in East London; and an old workhouse in Yorkshire offering modern medicine in a sub-standard setting.

There was and there always will be more to do.

The additional funding

This chapter is about how we managed the additional funding. It starts by looking at how we focussed the money on priorities and on reducing inequalities. It continues with an account of overall expenditure, including the use of private finance, and examines productivity and international comparisons.

The focus on priorities

The NHS Plan set out priorities and earmarked specific sums of additional money to be allocated to the NHS for them. Earmarking seems very logical but had some unfortunate side effects. The main one was that it led to a concentration on whether or not the money was actually being spent and not on whether the desired outcome was being achieved.

In cancer, for example, an extra £570 million a year was earmarked at the time of the NHS Plan for development. All the relevant interest groups – cancer clinicians, patients groups, politicians and the media – wanted to be able trace it and see whether it had been spent and whether it was truly over and above what would have been spent anyway by the NHS. This was difficult to prove and analysis and debate rumbled on over the next few years with claim and counter claim about what had actually happened.

Managers saw this as just plain unhelpful: earmarking £570 million or a bit more than 1% of the £49 billion total NHS expenditure in 2001/2 and tracing it through the 100 or so organisations which managed some cancer services was a time consuming additional task. More fundamentally they resisted any earmarking as they wanted maximum flexibility to spend their budgets over the entire range of activities so as to achieve the greatest synergy and efficiency. Most fundamentally of all, they wanted to be measured on outputs and outcomes and argued that if they could achieve the results for lower expenditure they should be praised – and not, as might happen, be criticized for underspending!

At the time, however, the Government wanted to demonstrate the impact of their policies and would send out press releases about how much money they were spending in health or education or elsewhere. It was too early to see actual results so extra spending was the measure they chose to demonstrate their achievements.

The truth was that we were all also trapped in our history in which extra money had been given to health and other services in the past and simply been dissipated by spending small amounts across the whole range of activities or used to deal with long standing problems or debts. History showed that the Government and cancer lobby were right to have suspicions about what might happen without monitoring.

It took some time for the Government to move on from this approach and they never did so fully. Ministers like announcing initiatives and extra bits of money for this or that. In the end it was counterproductive. The NHS and the public grew cynical. Announcements were seen as a substitute for action and all "new" money was assumed to be simply "double counting" the old.

Everything in health is a priority for someone, but we needed to prioritise to have the most effect. However, areas which were not priorities at the time felt neglected and lobbied hard for funding. I recall this being particularly true of renal services and neurosciences in the early days. We countered this by trying to have a rolling set of priorities – as one area improved another could become a priority – and by trying to make sure the non-priorities didn't get worse in the meantime. We also attempted to make sure that local managers had some scope for local priorities to meet the different needs in different parts of the country.

This is the sort of problem that will be familiar to anyone running any health system, large or small, anywhere. There is no textbook right answer. A balance between national and local priorities and non-priorities needs to be struck in each situation and constantly reviewed and adjusted. It is part of the art of management rather than the science.

Later, rather than earmarking funds, we were able to use "payment by results" to steer change and reinforce priorities. We could, for example, set the tariff for a particular surgical procedure at a level which assumed that 90% of them were done as day cases and only 10% involved an over night stay. This provided a clear incentive to do more day surgery. Over time this mechanism has become more sophisticated and funding can more easily be used to give priority and incentivise desirable changes.

A new "best practice" tariff is being developed. The best current example appears to be where 14% of the payment for treatment of hip fractures is kept back by the payer, and only paid to those hospitals which can demonstrate they followed a 10 point "best practice" protocol.

The Department could also promote priorities by adjusting the allocation of funds to the different parts of the country. Budgets were allocated to Health Authorities and PCTs on the basis of "weighted capitation" via a formula independently created by a working party led from the University of York which made recommendations to the Secretary of State on changes every three years. This formula was weighted to reflect the age of a particular population but also took account of its socio-economic and health status. It was then adjusted for the costs of providing services in the different areas.[1]

Each recalculation of the formula produced significant differences from the previous one, if for no other reason than that population sizes had changed in the intervening years. This led to adjustments that gave more funds to some parts of the country than others. For decades the Department had been working to create more and better services outside London with the particular ambition to get more specialist care to the north of the country where there was greater morbidity and life expectancy was lowest. As part of the NHS Plan reforms new cardiac units were opened, for example, in Blackpool and Wolverhampton and a new cancer centre built in Hull.

Each recalculation of the formula reinforced this trend so that by 2003 the poorest and sickest parts of the country received almost twice as much per head of the population as the wealthiest, even though costs for delivering services were much higher in the latter areas. Arguably this was the most effective thing we could do to help tackle inequalities in health.

This formula also has a political aspect. A Government can ask the working party to give more or less weight to particular factors such as deprivation. The Labour Government increased this weighting so that more funds flowed to poorer areas with greater levels of disease. The Coalition Government has reduced the deprivation weighting and redirected some of the money back to more affluent areas. It is perfectly legitimate for government to decide how much to weight deprivation but it does have obvious political implications and must be completely transparent.

The levels of funding

The new money started to flow into the NHS in 2001. Real term growth in the next 10 years averaged 5.5% a year as compared to the average over the previous 30 years of 3.9%.[*] Annual spend in cash terms more than doubled from £49 billion to £103 billion during this period. The biggest increase was in the five years between 2002/03 and 2007/08 when the additional funding agreed as a result of the Wanless Review resulted in an average real term growth of 7.4%.[2]

Table 8.1 shows average planned and real growth rates over different periods in the last 30 years. Three things stand out. The first is to see how surprisingly high growth has been throughout this period. The second is the astonishing boost that was given to the NHS in the last decade. The third is to see how little growth is planned over the next four years, with a real terms reduction in capital spend, albeit from a level more than double what it had been in 2001/02.

Financial management – and the rush for delivery

This massive growth fuelled expansion and improvement with the very large increases in staff and facilities and the service improvements described in earlier chapters. It was accompanied by a *rush for delivery*.

Implementation got off to a slow start as the NHS organised and mobilised. The result was that the political and public pressure to see improvement led to some of the initial spending being on more staff and more buildings rather than being invested more slowly on changed roles and new designs. Some managers simply "bought" improvements and falls in waiting lists. Early success was, as we have seen, sometimes measured in money spent not results achieved.

---

* *Real term* here means the amount left after the Treasury's GDP deflator – a measure of inflation – is taken off the full amount. In 2002/03, for example, NHS total expenditure grew by 10.2% but in real terms by only 6.8%.

Table 8.1 NHS Expenditure: England – average annual growth rates for key periods.

	Revenue Real Terms Growth	Capital Real Terms Growth	Total Real Terms Growth
1 Year Period – Plan (2011/12)	0.4%	−15.6%	−0.4%
2 Year Period – Plan (2011/12 to 2012/13)	0.3%	−9.1%	−0.1%
3 Year Period – Plan (2011/12 to 2013/14)	0.3%	−7.0%	−0.1%
4 Year Period – Plan (2011/12 to 2014/15)	0.2%	−4.8%	0.0%
5 Year Period – historical (2006/07 to 2010/11)	3.7%	14.8%	4.0%
10 Year Period – historical (2001/02 to 2010/11)	5.3%	11.9%	5.5%
15 Year Period – historical (1996/97 to 2010/11)	5.0%	5.0%	5.0%
20 Year Period – historical (1991/92 to 2010/11)	4.9%	4.0%	4.8%
15 Year Period – historical (1996/97 to 2010/11)	5.0%	5.0%	5.0%
20 Year Period – historical (1991/92 to 2010/11)	4.9%	4.0%	4.8%

This rush for delivery was probably inevitable but together with the impact of reorganisations and other factors meant that less attention was given to financial management. Financial pressures built up over the first few years of implementation as we rushed to improve services and meet targets. Activity increased as new facilities came on line and more people were recruited to staff them. The overspending on the Consultant and GP contracts added costs that hadn't been budgeted for.

In addition there was a particular problem which relates more generally to competition within the public sector. We have already seen in Chapter 5 that there was a political resistance to facing up to the fact that we had too much capacity in the NHS and that increased use of the private sector would lead to some closures of facilities. In practice some Trusts staffed up and opened new developments in anticipation of gaining more business from patient choice and competition; none contracted in anticipation of lost patient flows and income.

Organisations that take this sort of risk in the private sector are better able to manage the downside by laying off staff, closing facilities or even becoming bankrupt and walking away. NHS and other public sector organisations have fewer options – one reason, of course, why they are often more risk averse. Private sector organisations generally also have more experience at assessing risk than NHS Boards and Chief Executives – most of whom appeared to think they would be winners.

During this period there were varying numbers of up to 600 local NHS organisations – primarily Trusts, PCTs, and Health Authorities – which each had their own budgets and statutory accounts. These were all consolidated into a single NHS set of accounts. Some performed better financially than others. The performance management approach from "star ratings" to direct intervention was designed to ensure that all were able to manage their budgets – and if they didn't that they had credible recovery plans to do so.

We also, however, had to achieve balance across the NHS as a whole and ensure that organisational surpluses outweighed deficits.

By 2005/06 the financial pressures combined to defeat the normal processes for achieving balance and the NHS had a revenue deficit of £½ billion. Whilst this was less than 1% of revenue it was a material amount and the problems were spread around many NHS organisations which had both in year deficits and longer term debts.

Although I retired at this time for different reasons, as described in the next chapter; my leaving nevertheless allowed Sir Ian Carruthers and subsequently David Nicholson to come in as Chief Executive with a mandate to sort out the finances. They duly did so, creating a surplus of £½ billion the following year and £1.7 billion in the one afterwards. The large majority of NHS organisations got themselves into balance. It was a timely shock to the system that took some of the pressure out that had built over the previous five years in our rush for delivery.

As the flow of extra money stopped David once again gave a shock to the system by demanding that the NHS save £20 billion to meet cost pressures and to re-invest in new models of services. It is the sort of challenge that is needed to help bring about change. It is essential that the current Government follows it through with a vision of a new NHS and a strategy and plans for getting there.

Private finance

The NHS spent more than £28 billion on capital between 2001/02 and 2010/11 but also made extensive use of the Private Finance Initiative (PFI). £12.687 billion of private funding since 1997 is recorded as being allocated to 107 hospital projects completed, underway or being negotiated at March 2011.[3] They range in size from about £10 million to the £1 billion being spent at Barts and The London Hospitals. PFI was the biggest funder by far of major hospital developments whilst the NHS capital was used for a much wider range of equipment and smaller developments.

PFI had been started under the previous Conservative Government in order to increase capital spending in public projects over and above what was available from Government and as an attempt to introduce more discipline into public sector capital development. There were potential other benefits to be had from including estates maintenance and other hotel-type facilities in the contract.

The Treasury stated that the intended benefits of using PFI include:

- transferring the risk of failing to deliver services to time and budget to the private sector
- the maintenance of assets over the life of the contract
- transparency of service provision cost and
- innovative approaches to building design and service provision.[4]

This approach was built on a history in which a number of projects across the public sector had been badly specified at the outset, poorly managed during construction and been delivered very late and very over budget. The NHS had also suffered from a shortage of capital which limited its ability to adapt and change in line with service needs. Major capital projects had a high opportunity cost with the construction of the Chelsea and Westminster Hospital in west London in the early 90s, for example, consuming almost London's entire NHS capital budget for several years. The NHS estate had also, as we saw in the last chapter, suffered from lack of maintenance – often because these budgets were cut and the money transferred to direct patient care.

PFI seemed to promise a great deal; but it started very slowly in the early 90s because lenders and the NHS alike were cautious and inexperienced in working together. When Labour came into Government in 1997 they moved quickly to pass the NHS (Private Finance Act) 1997, which gave lenders greater comfort that their loans would be honoured, and prioritised a list of 20 developments for PFI.

At its simplest, PFI can be thought of as contract with a private supplier who takes out a loan to build a development to the client's specification, maintain it for typically 30 years and provide some other defined services such as cleaning. The client pays a sum of money each year to the contractor and, typically, at the end of the period owns the property. In some ways it is like a domestic mortgage in which the contractor builds and services the house.

The complexities come in the bidding process through which contractors are selected and in the detail of the contractual negotiations between prime contractors, subcontractors, lenders and client. In the early days these were very difficult and very lengthy indeed. There were some very problematic cases. The Norfolk and Norwich Hospital development, the first University Teaching Hospital to be built since the Second World War, was refinanced at a £116 million profit by its private funders who had taken a risk on currency transactions as part of the deal. The NHS received 29% of the profit but was exposed to a great deal of criticism as a result.[5] On the other side of the equation private contractors lost an equivalent amount in the development of Dudley Hospital.

Over time, however, the various different parties learned to work together and standard contracts and arrangements were developed. The process became much smoother. The volatility seen in Norfolk and Norwich and Dudley wasn't repeated.

The NHS Plan announced the extension of PFI into primary and community care through Local Improvement Finance Trusts (LIFT). These innovative structures brought investors and the NHS together into partnerships which worked locally by "batching" together a number of local low cost schemes to gain economies of scale. A number of LIFT partnerships have been very successful, whilst others have taken time to establish and make an impact.

PFI has been viewed as controversial throughout its history. In part this has undoubtedly been because of a widespread fear that it represented privatisation of the NHS and that the private sector would unfairly exploit access to public assets. The Norfolk and Norwich experience seemed to some critics to bear this out; although subsequent contracts have not.

More substantial criticism has been about whether or not the NHS was getting value for money for these deals or whether just taking a loan from Government or a bank would have been a cheaper option. It would certainly have been an easier one if it had eliminated some of the contractual process. However, others would argue that it was all the rigours of the contracting process, with its requirements to be clear about specifications, which brought some of the benefits in timely building processes and no cost over-runs. PFI, its proponents would argue, has introduced the necessary disciplines.

There is no clear way of deciding this argument. Each PFI scheme has to show that it is better value than a public sector comparator as part of the approval process; although the calculation depends on how whole life costs are calculated and on untestable assumptions about inflation. There is little scope for direct comparisons because so little was built with public capital over these years. The National Audit Office's cautious assessment in June 2010 after considering these issues was that:

> "We found that most PFI hospital contracts are well managed. And the low level of deductions and high levels of satisfaction indicate they are currently achieving the value for money expected at the point the contracts were signed." [6]

PFI really represented the only option for Chief Executives and Boards if they were going to able to rebuild their hospital, move from unfit and expensive to run old premises to new purpose built ones or expand their services. Some of them have very much welcomed the discipline the process brought.

Current concerns in the NHS are that the contracts are very inflexible when it comes to making post-contract changes in buildings or facilities and that the annual payments hospitals make to their PFI partners are so high as to be damaging future viability. There is some truth in both points. However, any new development, however funded, would cost a great deal to run and adapt. Capital isn't free and hospitals built with public money also face the same sorts of capital and other charges. The National Audit Office study identified no differences in value for money between services run by PFI partners or hospitals themselves.[7]

It is also worth looking at the figures. The National Audit Office recorded that the total cost to NHS Trusts of these annual payments in April 2009 was £890 million.[8] This figure includes some costs of estates and facilities management. It was less than 1% of NHS revenue at the time. The Department of Health has told me that as new schemes come on line this may rise to 2 to 3% of annual revenue. In broad terms this doesn't seem a damagingly high sum to be paying for all the new buildings and the various services attached to them.

Public finance

The trade was not all one way. The Department used public capital to invest outside the NHS through the LIFT schemes and otherwise. During these years we bought a failing London private hospital to expand capacity and an American blood company to safeguard supplies of plasma at a time when there were fears over the contamination of UK supplies.

We also set up a Joint Venture with Xansa in April 2005 to provide back office services. This, the brainchild of the Department's Director General of Finance Richard Douglas, has now developed so that it has more than 100 NHS organisations contracted for finance and accounting services.

Productivity

In almost any major investment and reform programme you would expect to see productivity fall initially as costs increase before the results are seen. This was anticipated with the NHS Plan. Moreover, costs were expected to rise in many cases as the NHS "caught up" with other countries. However, as we have seen, the "rush for delivery" meant in some cases that money was spent wastefully. It is therefore worth trying to understand what was achieved with the new money and how the improvements made compared with improvements made in other countries.

This is another complex and contested area. One approach is to look at productivity. Improving productivity at its simplest is about getting more for your money. It is about the ratio of outputs to inputs so that, for example, productivity can be improved either by getting more outputs for the same level of money or the same level of outputs for less money or a combination of these. It can be difficult to measure inputs but the main problem in health is how to measure the outputs, as the following examples show.

How can we factor in prevention of disease? Productivity in a hospital could be seen to rise because failures in community care meant that more patients were admitted as emergencies – hospital activity might go up with only marginal additional costs. Conversely, good preventative community care which kept people at home might mean hospital productivity went down.

How can we take quality into account? Is a better outcome for the patient a relevant factor in measuring productivity? What about safety or the length of waiting for treatment? The wrong measure will prioritise volume over quality and may produce perverse incentives. This is not just an issue for health or the public sector. It also applies to manufacturers who replace a cheaper model with a higher cost and higher quality product.

Many people have considered these issues, including Derek Wanless in reviewing the impact of his recommendations.[9] There is, however, no agreement about the best measures. Indeed, reading a cross section of media stories, audit reports and academic articles produces only confusion. Results vary depending on what measures are being taken – hospital productivity, Consultant productivity or whole system productivity – and the assessment seems to be heavily influenced by the views of the author.

I am not immune to such bias; but would suggest that a number of reputable bodies have tended towards a similar analysis that productivity fell by perhaps 1 to 1.5% a year during the early years of the plan as we expanded fast but was flat or even improving in the later years as results started to flow. There is an intuitive logic to this and it is what most economists would probably expect. It also reflects the reality of a period of "catch up" in resourcing.

Table 8.2 shows three different calculations. The first by the Office for National Statistics (ONS) makes no adjustment for any quality improvements. It shows productivity falling throughout the period. The second and third by the ONS and the Centre for Health Economics at York University (CHE) both make some adjustment for quality and produce the picture of falling productivity followed by flattening out.

These overall assessments of productivity are of limited value but offer some insight into the impact of the reforms. However, it is very important to be constantly searching for improved productivity when looking at individual processes or systems such as operating theatre utilisation, staff rotas and wastage levels. Some thinkers are now advocating that we should try to measure value in terms of a patient health outcome in relation to total cost.[10]

Year	1	2	3
	ONS HCHS Productivity (no quality adjustment)	ONS NHS Productivity (inc quality)	CHE NHS Productivity (inc quality)
1998/99	−0.6%	−0.3%	
1999/00	0.1%	0.2%	−2.7%
2000/01	−1.3%	−0.1%	−0.7%
2001/02	−0.6%	0.3%	−2.2%
2002/03	−4.7%	−1.9%	−1.2%
2003/04	−2.8%	−1.1%	−2.5%
2004/05	−1.5%	0.0%	−0.1%
2005/06	−1.4%	0.4%	1.6%
2006/07	−0.2%	1.0%	0.4%
2007/08	−1.6%	−0.4%	1.4%
AVERAGE	−1.5%	−0.2%	−0.7%

Table 8.2 Changes in productivity, as measured by ONS and CHE.

Ideally you would want to be able to assess the actual change experienced by a patient or a community as a result of a particular intervention or programme. Following a hip operation, for example, is a patient more mobile, able to do a wider range of things, return to work, be free from pain and so on? This sort of information is now available routinely from the Patient Reported Outcome Measures (PROMS) surveys.[11] It will allow the calculation of the actual change in patients' own views of their health status and hence the value of the operation to them.

John Appleby of the Kings Fund and colleagues are working on making this calculation. The results of their study are not yet published but John tells me that survey data shows that hip operations lead to very significant recorded improvements but there is a great deal of variation. One would expect hip operations to show good results as, anecdotally at least, they often seem to transform people's lives.

John also pointed out to me that being able to measure the health gain (outcomes) and the cost (inputs) of such an intervention would create a new measure of productivity, which would be of interest to clinicians and potentially bring them into effective dialogue with general and financial managers around outcomes and costs. This could be a very useful way forward.

International comparisons

Another way to look at productivity and the wider performance of the NHS is through making international comparisons. These comparisons, however, are only available for the UK as a whole – with England being about 85% of the population and slightly less of total UK spend.

Table 8.3 below shows spending on health as a percentage of GDP for seven countries with some similarities to the UK. It also shows how spend increased as a percentage of GDP over the NHS Plan period up to 2008, later figures are not yet available.

It shows that UK expenditure as a proportion of GDP remained the lowest throughout this period – despite the massive increase it received – with the possible exception of Australia (where 2008 figures aren't yet available). It also shows that the UK had only the fourth highest increase in this period with Australia and Germany controlling costs very tightly and the Netherlands and, predictably, the USA having the largest increases.

Most other western European countries increased their spending by between 1 and 2% of GDP during this period. The UK has still not caught up with the European average.[12]

The UK chose to increase its expenditure as part of a catch up and improvement process. None of these other countries had a comparably comprehensive plan during this period which aimed for improvement and reform in return for the growth. The increase in the US was simply market driven, with no national plan. This prompts the question as to whether the UK, with its intentional growth, was able as a result to improve its performance relative to the others.

There is limited evidence. The New York based Commonwealth Fund has done a series of broad based comparisons since 1999 and the UK has gradually performed better over this period. The latest publication, from which Figure 8.1 is taken, includes seven of the eight countries from Table 8.3 and shows the UK coming second in overall ranking to the Netherlands. The UK scores very highly – in the top two – on six of the 11 indicators: effective care, safe care, access, cost related problems, efficiency and equity. These are all extremely positive factors.

Table 8.3 Health spending by country and percentage of GDP[13]			
	% of **GDP** in 2000	% of **GDP** in 2008	Increase in % of GDP
UK	7.0	8.7	1.7
New Zealand	7.7	9.9	2.2
Australia	8.0	8.5 in 2007	0.5
Netherlands	8.0	9.9	1.9
Canada	8.8	10.4	1.6
France	10.1	11.2	1.1
Germany	10.3	10.5	0.2
USA	13.4	16.0	2.6

Figure 8.1 International comparisons of performance[14]

Exhibit ES-1. Overall Ranking

Country Rankings						
1.00-2.33						
2.34-4.66						
4.67-7.00						

	AUS	CAN	GER	NETH	NZ	UK	US
OVERALL RANKING (2010)	3	6	4	1	5	2	7
Quality Care	4	7	5	2	1	3	6
Effective Care	2	7	6	3	5	1	4
Safe Care	6	5	3	1	4	2	7
Coordinated Care	4	5	7	2	1	3	6
Patient-Centered Care	2	5	3	6	1	7	4
Access	6.5	5	3	1	4	2	6.5
Cost-Related Problem	6	3.5	3.5	2	5	1	7
Timelines of Care	6	7	2	1	3	4	5
Efficiency	2	6	5	3	4	1	7
Equity	4	5	3	1	6	2	7
Long, Healthy, Productive Lives	1	2	3	4	5	6	7
Health Expenditures/Capita, 2007	$3,357	$3,895	$3,588	$3,837*	$2,454	$2,992	$7,290

Note: *Estimate. Expenditures shown in $US PPP (purchasing power parity).
Source: Calculated by The Commonwealth Fund based on 2007 International Health Policy Survey; 2008 International Health Policy Survey of Sicker Adults; 2009 International Health Policy Survey of Primary Care Physicians; Commonwealth Fund Commission on a High Performance Health System National Scorecard; and Organization for Economic Cooperation and Development, OECD Health Data, 2009 (Paris: OECD, Nov. 2009). Reproduced with permission from The Commonwealth Fund.

It scores in the bottom two on two indicators: patient centred care and long, healthy, productive lives. Both are vitally important. The second seems to be related to relatively poor management of risks factors for heart disease and cancer and subsequent treatment. Whilst there have been improvements here and a wider study of mortality amenable to healthcare shows the UK making some comparative improvement, it is still a very long way behind the leaders on these aspects.[15]

In assessing the overall performance of the NHS in England during this period, it is also important to look at the findings of its own independent regulator, the Healthcare Commission, and the comparison with the other three countries of the UK which also had the same increases in funding but did not have the NHS Plan.

The Healthcare Commission in 2008 concluded that "*the NHS has made some dramatic progress*" and drew attention to improvements from waiting times to mental health and reducing smoking. It also commented on the persistence of inequalities in health outcomes and the risks from obesity and non-communicable diseases which had emerged as the major problems for the future.[16] Another independent report from the Nuffield Trust also identified significant improvements and drew attention to the need for a greater focus on quality and not just volume of activity.[17]

Very significantly a review of improvement in the four countries of the UK – England, Scotland, Wales, and Northern Ireland – which had all received the same increases in funding showed that England had outperformed all the others by a considerable margin.[18]

Most tellingly of all, as we have already noted, public satisfaction doubled, patients returned from the private sector and all the political parties now support the NHS.

Sustainability

The enormous boost in funding helped "*save*" the NHS. However, as Table 8.1 shows us the NHS has had average real terms rises of 3.9% for the last 30 years. Even during the decline in the 80s and 90s average growth was around 3%. Yet it has virtually no growth planned for the next four years.

This is the size of the sustainability problem that will be addressed when we look at the future in Chapter 12.

Conclusions and key points

1. There always need to be priorities in health. Financial measures and *payment by results* can ensure they get attention; whilst financial allocations can be used to deliver funding to the poorest and least healthy populations in the country.

2. By 2006 the "rush for delivery", new facilities and staff becoming available and the pressures of competition led to a build up of financial pressure in the system and to the NHS overspending. The NHS returned to surplus the following year but is now facing severe financial difficulty with virtually no real term growth for the next four years.

3. The Private Finance Initiative was the major funder of hospital developments with over £12 billion invested and more committed to LIFT for community and primary care premises. After early problems, the NHS and its partners learned how to manage the process effectively and have delivered many fine new buildings. The PFI capital has to be paid for in annual instalments which may eventually amount to 2 to 3% of annual spend. Similar levels of costs would have been incurred by any capital programme.

4. There are no generally agreed ways of assessing the productivity of a health system like the NHS and there are particular difficulties in accounting for prevention work and quality improvements. The best available measures which take some account of quality gains suggest that productivity shrank by about 1.5% a year in the early years as the new funding flowed in and that it improved to a neutral position as the results appeared thereafter. There appear to be some new and promising ways of measuring the actual value of health gained through particular interventions.

Conclusions and key points (*Continued*)

5. Despite the massive increases in the NHS budget UK health spending is still lower than almost all its main comparator countries. Many of them had similar levels of increased funding over this period, although none appears to have had the same planned investment as part of a development strategy.

6. The UK's performance improved relative to most other comparator countries during this period. The NHS in England, which alone implemented the NHS Plan, significantly outperformed the other UK countries during this period.

7. The independent Healthcare Commission identified "*some dramatic progress*" as well as areas like inequalities and obesity to concentrate on for the future.

References

1. Department of Health (2003) *Resource allocation: Weighted Capitation Formula*; 31 March.
2. Derek Wanless (2002) *Our future health: taking a long-term view*; HM Treasury, April.
3. Department of Health website.
4. National Audit Office (2010) *The performance and management of hospital PFI contracts*; June, para 1.1, p 12.
5. House of Commons: *The re-financing of the Norfolk and Norwich PFI Hospital*; Parliamentary Accounts Committee 35th Report session 2005–06.
6. National Audit Office (2010) *The performance and management of hospital PFI contracts*; June, Summary para 18, p 8.
7. Ibid.
8. Ibid. para 1.2, p 12.
9. Derek Wanless, John Appleby, Anthony Harrison, Darshan Patel (2007) *Our future secured? A review of NHS funding and performance*; Kings Fund, p 18.
10. Kim JY, Rhatigan J, Jain SH, Weintraub R, Porter ME (2010) From a declaration of values to the creation of value in global health: a report from Harvard University's Global Health Delivery Project. *Glob Public Health* **5**: 181–8.
11. Department of Health (2009) *PROMS questionnaires: terms and conditions*; 29 April.
12. From OECD: *Health data* 2010; version October 2010.
13. Ibid.
14. The Commonwealth Fund: *Mirror, mirror on the wall: how the performance of the US health system compares internationally, 2010 update*.
15. Nolte E, McKee CM (2008) Measuring the health of nations: updating an earlier analysis. *Health Affairs* **27**(1): 58–71.
16. The Healthcare Commission: state of healthcare in England and Wales; 2008, p5.
17. Leatherman S, Sutherland K (2008) *The quest for quality in the NHS: refining the NHS reforms*. Nuffield Trust.
18. Connolly S, Bevan G, Mays N (2010) *Funding and performance of healthcare systems in the UK before and after devolution*. Nuffield Trust.

Chapter 9

Leadership

When I was Chief Executive of the Oxford Radcliffe I appointed clinical directors in every speciality. Almost all were doctors. They took on what I think is one of the most difficult roles in healthcare. Each was expected to provide leadership for their whole service and, with support from a business manager, deliver the annual plan and manage the budget.

It was a tough role. I remember one of them telling me that he had woken up in the night in a sweat because he had dreamed that I had asked him to secure peace in Northern Ireland and he wasn't sure how he was going to do it.

"I hope you felt better when you woke up." I said soothingly.

"No I didn't", he replied, *"I found that you had persuaded me to take on neo-natal intensive care."*

This book contains many stories of people like Peter who stepped out of their normal role and their comfort zone in order to try to make things better. I have endless admiration for the many people – managers as well as clinicians – who were willing to take the risk of being leaders in often very difficult circumstances. Mostly they succeeded.

Leadership

The whole success of the service redesign I described in Chapter 4 depended on hundreds of people choosing to take a lead. Looking more widely at the NHS, there are literally thousands of leaders, all of whom influence in some way the care of patients and the motivation and morale of staff.

This chapter starts with local leadership in the NHS and describes something of its complications and pressures. It moves on to the national picture and considers the role that national institutions play before looking at the relationship between the political and managerial processes and describing how we forged a "guiding coalition" which served us very well for three years from 2002.

I also take a few pages to discuss my own role as Chief Executive of the NHS and Permanent Secretary of the Department of Health where I had both managerial responsibilities and worked closely with Ministers on policy. I describe the way in which I tried to make this work, not always successfully, by keeping a focus on delivery whilst building relationships with many of the key people in the NHS and beyond.

Local leadership in the NHS

Clinicians – doctors, nurses and others – are the natural leaders in the NHS and many of the most senior spend a great deal of their time organising and shaping services at the most local levels. Some take on wider clinical director, nursing director and medical director roles. Doctors in particular, can find this transition very difficult.

Almost all doctor/managers continue at least part time with their clinical role and, mostly, will return to it full time after a spell as clinical director or in some leadership role for their practice, PCT or GP Consortium. In the meantime, however, they may well have to make themselves unpopular and to persuade some of their colleagues to change their work patterns or to conform to organisational or NHS policies. They may even have to speak to them about their behaviour of give them feedback on clinical or other performance issues.

This is very difficult territory. I recall, for example, one Consultant telling me that he was trying to deal with a difficult colleague who was not doing his share of the work and whose whole approach to the job was idiosyncratic and inconsistent. He didn't get any support from his Medical Director and found himself facing a formal grievance procedure for alleged harassment. Eventually he won but it was a difficult and frustrating time. I know of other such examples but happily they are rare. Nevertheless a doctor who signs up for a management role may well find that colleagues think that he or she has "gone over to the dark side".

At Oxford the Medical and Nursing Directors and I worked very closely together in order to make sure we had a seamless approach to these issues and, although we didn't describe it like this at the time, to provide role models for the hospital and demonstrate the behaviour we wanted to see.

I also re-learned at Heatherwood and Wexham and in Oxford something that I knew from other sectors: that there are many sorts of leadership roles in an organisation. This is perhaps particularly true in healthcare where each of the tribes – the nurses, doctors, pharmacists, therapists, scientists and so on – have their leaders; so does each ward and department and all the professional bodies, trades unions and social societies.

There are also the rather special people in a hospital who know everyone, who pass on news or gossip, who connect different areas together and can be amongst the greatest influencers and informal leaders in the whole place. I have seen switchboard operators, the senior theatre sister, the Board Secretary and others play this sort of role. Chaplains can be very important because they see patients and staff, often at very traumatic times and frequently have very good knowledge about what is going on in a hospital.

When most or all these groups line up in the same direction they can be very powerful indeed. A wise Chief Executive, I learned, understood who these many leaders were, stayed in touch with them and, wherever possible, worked with them to make changes happen.

I was also reminded that people were motivated at work by many different things, some quite personal, but that almost everyone I met from the porter and cleaner to the doctor and physiotherapist was motivated by, to some extent, wanting to get it right for the patient in front of them. This was partly a human response to pain and suffering: of wanting to help and knowing that you can make a difference in the lives of individuals whether with friendliness and comfort or clinical skills and technical expertise.

For many people there is also a personal and professional pride in using skills and knowledge, solving problems and doing so to the highest standards. I remember one Friday meeting a scientist in a Public Health Laboratory Service facility in Yorkshire. There is a rare genetic condition which puts women seriously at risk during pregnancy and requires close monitoring. This was the only laboratory that tested for the problem and he was the only scientist that did the test. At any one time he was keeping weekly track of about 20 women as they progressed through pregnancy. They never knew he existed; but he was silently cheering them on through their term and was delighted when they made it through to a safe delivery. His passion and commitment equalled anything I saw from the clinicians who worked directly with patients.

Healthcare can be very rewarding with the knowledge that you have made a difference – even when patients don't know you exist – although often, of course, patients and relatives express their grateful thanks. Many clinicians also get an enormous amount of satisfaction out of doing things better than others, of being amongst the best in their particular field and of receiving professional recognition. There is a mix here of selflessness and ego. On occasions, of course, there is much more ego than selflessness.

Policy makers can make the mistake of thinking that financial incentives are enough to motivate people. My observation is that such incentives can change behaviour but they rarely motivate. The new Consultant contract was a case in point. It changed the way things were done but was resented by many doctors who thought it demeaned them and their contribution. It de-motivated rather than motivated.

A policy paper I wrote in 2005 identified the main motivators for individuals, teams and organisations, listing such factors as personal altruism, patients' responses both face to face and through surveys, professional autonomy and feedback from inspection. It argued that all these motivators needed to be aligned in the NHS and with partners outside to achieve the greatest success.[1]

Many people in the NHS have very strong motivational ties to their own patients, their own services and their own hospital or practice. Many also have an emotional connection to the values and to the whole concept of the NHS. Their link to the particular organisation where they work – the Trust or the PCT – is often much weaker. It is contingent on how the organisation behaves, how they are treated and what relationships its leaders build with them.

It is all too easy for the natural local leaders to be disengaged from the wider organisation, to keep their head down and to carry on with their work and ignore national and regional issues. Serial re-organisation and the high turnover of senior managers in some areas didn't help. I found a sense in some places that was almost as if the NHS was an occupied territory – perhaps like Southern Italy over the centuries – where waves of different invaders in the form of Governments and managers came through, stayed a while, left a few traces behind them and were in turn overwhelmed by the next wave. The inhabitants meanwhile found the best way to survive under each of the different invaders and carried on as far as possible with their normal patterns of behaviour.

This is a caricature, of course, but it does illustrate the importance of finding ways to engage these natural leaders in the wider enterprise in order to help make improvements at a large scale. This issue of engagement particularly of doctors is important for all health systems and there is an extensive literature written about it. Over the NHS reform years we tried many ways of building and sustaining engagement including the appointment of national clinical directors as well as local ones, funding training programmes and providing support for organisations like the British Association of Medical Managers which championed these links. Some progress was made.

The corollary of this problem is that when clinicians do engage and are given their head they can be very effective as earlier examples show – from Keith Willett and Peter Worlock transforming the trauma service in Oxford, to George Alberti leading a national "movement" in emergency care and the hundreds of GPs transferring roles to other staff. This, of course, was why our policy of appointing National Clinical Directors or Czars was so successful. These examples show what can be done and as a new generation of clinicians emerge who have some training in policy, management and leadership their leaders are already doing their own thinking, writing their own books on the subject and running their own learning sets.[2]

Chief Executives, managers and Non Executive Directors shared many of the characteristics of the clinicians and other staff. They, too, were generally motivated by patients and by making a difference – it was why most of us joined the NHS in the first place. It was also why many Non Executives became involved: to "do something for the local community" or "give something back". Some, me included, became fiercely attached to our institutions. As a rule, however, I think that most directors and managers had a wider perspective on the NHS than other staff, had wider loyalties and recognised their role in contributing to the NHS as a whole.

There has been a great deal of controversy about the relationship between managers and clinicians. There are some broad differences between the two groups in perspective and thinking. Clinicians will often be concerned more with individual patients, managers with the population. In my observation clinicians tend to be more concrete thinkers dealing with the detail and the here and now whilst managers will be more abstract and look at patterns. These differences leave great scope for misunderstandings and tension.

In practice there are many examples of excellent working relationships between clinicians and managers where both bring something distinctive to their joint endeavour. I have heard many clinicians criticise managers in general but then say "*but we are lucky, we have a good one who understands what needs to be done*".

There were, of course, some poor managers and plenty of poor relationships between clinicians and managers. This was not always the managers' fault. Part of our task at the centre was to provide training and development and to replace the poor ones. As often, however, it was to provide the support managers needed in introducing difficult changes. Sometimes leaders and managers need to be unpopular.

I learned a great deal working in three NHS organisations in the 80s and 90s about how the NHS really worked, who the leaders were, what motivated people and what we as managers could and couldn't do. It stood me in good stead when I moved to the national role.

Local leadership – NHS Boards

Chairs, Non Executive Directors and Boards play a very important role in the NHS in providing local leadership for organisations and holding the executives to account. I was privileged to work with two excellent Boards as a Trust Chief Executive and know how much the experience of Non Executives from outside can offer and what a Board can do to provide leadership and direction as well as secure the future of the organisation.

This isn't, however, universally the case. As NHS Chief Executive with oversight of as many as 600 NHS organisations I have seen the full range from those that resisted taking any responsibility – blaming everything on politicians or the Department – to those which turned round failing organisations through their own efforts.

The NHS has been on a long journey with its Boards from the inception of the first NHS Trusts in 1991. During the NHS Plan period Sir William Wells, Chairman of the independent Appointments Commission which appointed most Non Executives, set out a framework for improving governance within NHS Boards which stressed their responsibilities and accountabilities. He also led a series of training programmes and conferences with Chairs and Non Executives to help develop both their understanding of the issues and their capabilities.

Monitor, too, has played an important role in improving Boards by assessing their governance capabilities – and rejecting some – as part of its authorisation process for Foundation Trusts.

Governance at the local as well as the national level is challenged by the Mid Staffordshire Inquiry – how was such abuse and neglect allowed to continue unnoticed for so long – and will come under increasing pressure as the NHS adapts to the current financial climate. Boards, however, are likely to have an increasingly important role to play in a more decentralised and local NHS which needs to work more effectively with local partners.

Leadership nationally – national institutions

I described in Chapter 2 the way that the big national institutions of healthcare, the universities and commerce all play a significant part in shaping the health environment – sometimes for the greater good and sometimes in their own interests. They were able to wield a lot of political and financial power. This was evident both at the local level and nationally.

Locally, I think that these national influences were often restrictive. People couldn't do things because of Royal College rules or so as not to break solidarity with the profession or because they had a long term relationship with a University. In a similar vein I described earlier how patterns of private practice could interfere with NHS planning.

Nationally, it was more mixed. Royal College Presidents, Medical School leaders and voluntary organisations' Chief Executives in particular played a very significant role in helping develop the NHS Plan. They were often able to speak independently and therefore carried greater weight with the public and politicians than NHS leaders could.

Leadership nationally – the political dimension

For 5 years the Secretary of State of the time and I met with the Prime Minister almost every fortnight. Perhaps 20 times a year we came to the Cabinet Room or more informally to his office in Number 10 or to Chequers, his official country residence, to discuss the NHS.

They were surprisingly managerial meetings. He wanted to know about the latest progress with targets and what the obstacles were and to discuss tactics as well as strategy. Mostly these were challenging but constructive and energising meetings where we spoke frankly and shared ideas. I remember one occasion, however, in late 2001 which was rather different.

We were seated at the Cabinet Table. The Prime Minister and his advisers on one side: the Secretary of State and myself on the other flanked by our teams. Money was being spent but results weren't coming: waiting lists stayed high and public scepticism about the possibility of improvement was rising. The Prime Minister wasn't happy and demanded to know what I was going to do. "Yes," said the Secretary of State, "*what are you going to do?*" He and his entourage leaned back from the table, isolating me.

I did the only thing I could and leaned forward confidently, looked the Prime Minister in the eye and told him that things were beginning to change and that he would see the results starting to come through in the new year. He could trust me on this. I knew what was happening out there. I was grateful to David Fillingham, head of the Modernisation Agency, beside me who also leaned forward. I don't know if the Prime Minister believed me or not.

It was a tense moment which could have marked a damaging change in our relationships. In fact things started to improve just as and when I had said they would. It was also a vivid reminder of the high stakes we were playing for.

Funding the NHS Plan was a bold political act of will. There was a great deal of political as well as financial capital bound up in it. More importantly, the future of the NHS was at stake and with it the principles of healthcare available to all "*regardless of the ability to pay*".

The politics and politicians brought us many benefits. They were responsible for the enormous increase in money and for an input of energy and hope into a service that, despite the great efforts of its leaders of the time, was drifting and declining in the 90s. The high profile politics, the public focus and the media always on the look out for problems were all very irritating, but they kept the pressure up. The NHS could easily have settled for some of its early gains. It had often seen politicians arrive with a burst of energy on election. They made some progress but were distracted onto other issues by the second or third year. This was different: very high profile politics and the Prime Minister's own focus on health kept the pressure going year on year.

I recall a surgeon telling me in 2003 that his waiting list was now down to 6 months: that was surely good enough, wasn't it. No, it wasn't.

Politics, of course, also brought complications. These came in three areas. The first was the baggage of ideology, commitment and policy that governments bring with them into office. Much of what the Labour Government brought was beneficial to the NHS with a visceral support for its values and integrity. However, this support came with some very fixed ideas about, for example, all NHS services needing to be delivered by NHS organisations which led to great tensions within the Labour Party as *New* and *Old* fought it out.

Many of these tensions needed to be resolved within the political party and these internal struggles had relatively little impact on the NHS, but some overflowed into policy and management.

A classic example was *Agenda for Change* where the Government came into power with manifesto and other commitments to raising pay for NHS staff and increasing staffing levels and with some very close policy and personal ties with trades unions. This put enormous limitations on the manoeuvrability of the Department and NHS negotiators. Much had been given away before they even reached the table. The result was an overemphasis on targets for growth in staff numbers and staff members who had already discounted the increases they had been promised by Labour in opposition and now had even higher expectations.

This, of course, was simply part of the system for us. We had to get on with the cards we were dealt; knowing that any Government comes with its own views, allegiances and alliances. Even in countries where the health system has no direct connection with politics a government's role in legislation sets political boundaries around healthcare and shapes what happens in the country.

The second area was public and press relations: a central concern of any Government, which sometimes degenerated into "spin". The Government had set the agenda with the NHS Plan and wanted to maintain momentum with regular positive updates on progress and the announcement of new initiatives which showed it was in control of events. Initially, as we saw in the last chapter, it presented progress in terms of money spent because there weren't yet any results; although over time both the results and the announcements improved.

Many of its initiatives and announcements were designed to respond to or head off criticism and to rebut critics who said they weren't doing enough about X or failing on Y. Some were simply time consuming and distracting such as announcing that every ward sister would be given a budget to spend as they saw fit. It led to endless problems of identifying what this covered: was mental health included and five day wards; were wards which already had budgets included and so on? Others were very welcome by drawing attention to neglected areas such as learning disabilities or mental health.

There were two other deeper problems in this area. The first was the importance of maintaining trust and confidence in official statistics. We were very careful to keep definitions about what constituted a waiting list, admission to hospital or a hospital bed – as opposed to a trolley – the same as they had been for many years beforehand. We didn't want to be accused of choosing definitions that simply suited what we or the Government wanted to present. Over time the release of official statistics became more and more tightly controlled so that Ministers had little access to them before publication in order to remove any hint of political interference.

The second was that because the Government had identified itself so closely with the success of the NHS, the NHS in turn became seen as being too close to Government. It found itself being attacked for political reasons. Where one might have naively hoped that there would be some objective reporting of developments good or bad, virtually everything was politicised. There was little shared national pleasure in a new service or hospital opening but only an opportunity to make political capital. Politics and the media fed off each other.

This is not unique to the UK or to this particular Government, of course; but where a Government and a health system or health reform are so closely identified with Government – as in the US currently for example – most rational debate goes out the window. It was interesting to note that during much of this period patient and public satisfaction with the performance NHS locally rated much higher than satisfaction with the NHS nationally. The local figures appeared to be based on what people actually experienced whilst the national figures were more linked to support levels for the Government. Both figures rose during this period.

Similarly, people who had used the NHS recently rated it much higher than those who had only read about or heard about it from others. Pollsters heard comments like *"we are lucky locally but I know there are problems nationally"*. It was an echo of the clinicians' views about managers that I described earlier.

The third area concerned the level of involvement of politicians and their advisers in implementation and day to day operations. There is authoritative precedent here of course. Aneurin Bevan, who brought the NHS into existence, said that a bedpan dropped on an NHS ward would reverberate around Whitehall. Successive Secretaries of State certainly heard the sound. The most recent ones have employed people constantly to monitor the media for the echoes: sometimes so that they can rebut damaging stories and sometimes so that they can intervene.

My predecessors, successors and I have all discussed with our Secretaries of State where and when we should or should not intervene from the centre. I have taken many calls from Ministers and their advisers when the newspaper first editions come out just before midnight in which we have talked about local events and possible interventions. This was particularly frequent in the first few years when we were tackling "winter crises". It reduced over time as we decentralised power.

There were times, of course, when such interventions were useful because they sent powerful messages through the system about what the politicians saw as important. At other times the chief function of myself and other senior managers in the Department was to provide what became known as "air cover" – some protection for people in the NHS to get on with the job in hand without political interference.

Political or special advisers were first appointed by Harold Wilson with numbers increasing under Margaret Thatcher. They really became controversial, however, when Labour brought much larger numbers into much more powerful posts after 1997. They were widely seen as usurping the Civil Service's traditional role in policy development and providing advice to Ministers. Ministers on the other hand appear to see them as adding expertise to a largely generalist civil service and, perhaps more importantly, as providing political perspective and a very personal loyalty to their masters.

As I write there is once again debate about the future of our impartial Civil Service and questioning as to whether there needs to be a wider range of experience brought into it and, perhaps, more political appointments. My own observation is that wider experience may well be helpful but that it is vital to have a core of very experienced experts on Government at the centre: people who know what it was like when we had security, financial and other crises 20 years ago, who were there when it happened and have useful corporate and constitutional memory. They can add some balance and perhaps ballast to the decision making of the government of the day. It doesn't all have to be invented as they go along.

On political and special advisers, my very pragmatic view is that some were very able and added value whilst some were completely useless and just got in the way … with a whole range in between. Some made a big contribution: Simon Stevens, a young economist, worked closely with Alan Milburn on the writing of the Plan; Paul Corrigan, married to Cabinet Minister Hilary Armstrong, brought experience of politics and local government to the role; and, later, Julian Le Grand added academic economics to the mix. They were all very influential in policy development and political presentation and it was their influence, particularly Simon's, that gave the reform such an economic bias as opposed to a more business, managerial or clinical focus.

I discovered one unexpected bonus from these roles. Just as Departments found it was useful to have strong Ministers to fight the cross Whitehall battles and stand up to the Treasury, I discovered it was useful to have special advisers who could fight the cross Government political barriers. Advisers from the Civil Service couldn't do this. It was helpful to know that these advisers were locked in struggle with their peers in the Treasury at the same time as we argued, no doubt much more politely, with our colleagues in Whitehall about Foundation Hospitals and other controversial policies.

The final part of the mix was the various policy and monitoring units which were created at various times in Number 10 or the Treasury. I have commented on them earlier in Chapter 5 where I discussed system reform. The simple point to note here is that my colleagues worked closely with Sir Michael Barber as head of the Prime Minister's Delivery Unit from its creation in 2004 to make sure that we all had the same data and analysis.

It was enormously helpful to me to know that Michael was briefing the Prime Minister before our meetings with the same information as I had. It not only helped me to "manage up", as the expression goes, but undoubtedly also helped to build confidence in me and the Department.

The guiding coalition

Over time we created what I began to think of as a guiding coalition of politicians and Departmental leaders and established a very consistent way of working between ourselves. There were around 9 people in it at any time – the Prime Minister and his advisers, the Secretary of State and his advisers and me and a few senior colleagues. We knew what we were planning to do, we had the same data and we had developed a degree of trust between us.

This guiding coalition lasted from 2002 to the election in 2005 – the period of the most radical changes – and survived some important changes of personnel. The most risky was when John Reid replaced Alan Milburn as Secretary of State in 2003. Reid, like Milburn, was close to the Prime Minister and moved very easily into the role and maintained continuity of purpose. He was supported by John Hutton who had a leading role as Minister of State and was effectively the Secretary of State's deputy throughout this period. He had developed an enormous amount of knowledge and experience of the health and social care system after first being appointed to the Department as Minister for Social Care in 1998.

On the Department's side I was joined in this guiding coalition by Neil McKay and later John Bacon and Duncan Selbie as the Directors responsible for delivery and, on occasion, by Liam Donaldson and Chris Beasley as the Chief Medical Officer and Chief Nursing Officer respectively.

There were, of course, differences and tensions in this group as I have described in Chapter 5, for example, where I believed that politicians didn't face up to the consequences of involving the private sector. We didn't all agree all the time. However, my observation was that we had got to know each other well enough over this period and had sufficient shared experience to form a reasonably strong working relationship and sense of shared purpose. I believe that having this coherence at the top across the political managerial boundary was crucially important in enabling us to make so much change so quickly. Discord at this level would have slowed us down and might have derailed the Plan.

The guiding coalition fell apart after the 2005 election when all the senior politicians and advisers with the exception of the Prime Minister changed. We didn't build up the same relationships with the new ones during my time in the Department.

My role and approach

We all brought different things to the guiding coalition and came at it with our different perspectives and allegiances. When I was appointed in 2000 I had rather naively thought that I was joining a team of some sort where we had shared goals and were all essentially on the same side. I had a simple and rather unsophisticated management model in my head. I soon learned that this wasn't the case and that the idea of a temporary coalition of interests rather than a team was nearer the mark. There was sufficient overlap to agree on a shared direction most of the time but we all had different bottom lines and different long term goals.

I am often asked what it was like to work so closely with politicians and how I balanced my twin roles of Chief Executive and Permanent Secretary. There are a few simple pointers here which really apply to any job. The first was to understand the context fully in terms of the business, relationships and power and, within this, to be aware of the differing motivations of the different people. The second was to think about where there was common ground and who my best allies might be. The third was to be crystal clear about what it was that I personally brought to the party in terms of special skills or knowledge that others didn't have. The fourth and most easily overlooked was to make sure that others knew what my special contribution was – where I added value – over and above my job title and job description.

I was dealing with four different contexts – the political, the civil service, the NHS and social care – but tried generally to take the same approach to each of them. Having discussed politics and the NHS so far in this chapter I will spend a moment on the other two.

I joined the Civil Service when I became a Regional Director in 1997 and therefore had had some exposure to it before becoming the Permanent Secretary in 2000. The differences with the NHS were profound. Where the NHS was passionate, outward looking towards patients and focused on action; the Civil Service was dispassionate, looking upwards to support their Ministers and were interested in policy. It will be obvious from this account that I was more typical of the NHS than the Civil Service.

I gained a great deal from my Civil Service role and valued the opportunity to meet with the Cabinet Secretary and fellow Permanent Secretaries from all the other Departments at our Wednesday meetings. It helped put health into the wider context and to build bridges with education, sport and home affairs amongst others. I cultivated these relationships wherever appropriate. Some leverage in Whitehall was important. However, the NHS/Civil Service relationship was uncomfortable within the Department.

The Department had long been spilt between those looking outwards to the NHS and those looking upwards to Ministers. My two roles had been joined together to give maximum leverage at a time of great change and it was certainly very useful that I didn't have to negotiate with a peer all the time about resources, direction and personnel. However, I effectively made it for more than five years the *Department for the NHS* rather than the *Department of Health* and I know that some civil servants found this very difficult. I relied very heavily on Sir Hugh Taylor, who was later my successor as Permanent Secretary, to advise me on my role as Permanent Secretary and to be a leadership figure for the civil servants in the Department.

When I retired my recommendation that the roles be separated again was accepted. I have argued in the House of Lords and elsewhere that there needs to be far greater separation between the Department and the NHS, partly to allow the NHS to escape some of its political control but also to enable the Department to fulfil its role better in promoting health across the country and across Government.[3, 4]

The relationship between the NHS and social care was often also a strained one. The NHS was led and managed from within the Department. Social care, however, was the responsibility of Local Authorities. The Department provided policy leadership and supported the Inspector of Social Services. Social Services Directors and Local Authority Chief Executives often felt that they were treated poorly compared to the NHS and even neglected or forgotten about in our rush for delivery in the NHS.

There is a lot of truth in this. In some parts of the country the NHS and social care developed very strong relationships but elsewhere it was a fault line that caused problems for patients and staff alike. It was aggravated by a lack of consistency across different local authorities. All had the same duties but each could interpret or fund them in different ways and sometimes both local and national politics got in the way. Looking forward, as we shall do in the next few chapters, finding ways to bridge the gaps between the NHS and other local services will be one of the most essential contributors to continuing success.

Results and inclusiveness

I adopted very much the same approach in each of these four contexts by focusing on two things: results and inclusiveness. The first is, of course, obvious. I had been appointed to implement the NHS Plan and needed to make sure that results were delivered through the accountability and improvement processes I had established.

The second was rather more subtle. Health and healthcare are very broad areas with many different stakeholders and many different leaders. I took the view that I needed to work with as many as possible and to draw them into shared leadership: in a coalition as I described above, if not a team. I particularly focussed on Chief Executives and some Chairs in the NHS so as to make sure that we had a unified NHS approach; but I also worked with others including some patients' groups, the Presidents of the largest Royal Colleges and the Chief Executives of some Local Authorities.

This had a number of benefits. The main one, of course, was that it allowed us to align our efforts and our energies wherever we could. However, it also meant that I needed to understand the NHS and its people and partners in as much depth as possible. I cultivated relationships, visited extensively, read, listened and learned and within a short while knew the NHS across the country better than anyone else. This knowledge coupled with my relationship with Chief Executives gave me a natural power base and authority. When I met with Ministers or participated in the guiding coalition I was able to bring special knowledge and experience to the table.

Put more colloquially, I could out-anecdote the politicians who frequently came back from the House or their constituencies with tales of who they had talked with and what they had been told. I could often provide context and give them examples that were different from theirs or that confirmed their story. This was very important because policy or initiatives were sometimes created on the spot – sometimes even based only on one incident – and people or institutions got bad reputations because of a single story. I was able to head off some such problems.

In opting for these two approaches, results and inclusiveness, I necessarily eschewed others. Chief Executives can't do everything and need to rely on colleagues to fulfil many essential leadership roles. There are choices here. I didn't, for example, concentrate as much on policy as someone else might have done but relied on many excellent colleagues. I also didn't seek to make myself a public figure as others might have wanted to do. As a civil servant there were in any case limits to what I could say. In practice, Ministers largely occupied this space: although I and others did give interviews, make public statements and hold press conferences when we were the best people to do it. I, for example, fronted the twice annual reporting of results and dealt with many of the non-political criticisms of the NHS.

Like any Chief Executive I adopted an approach that suited me. I am very much action-orientated and prefer to get things done through engaging others. As with other experienced leaders I can and do adopt many different styles but these are my most natural ones.

Leadership nationally – the Department and the NHS

Early on I made it clear to Chief Executives that I wanted them and their organisations to behave as *One NHS*. I wanted to see partnerships and cooperation and I didn't want to see private disagreements erupting into the public arena. It was at a time when we were centralising the NHS to get the grip we needed for delivery.

As part of this I brought together over 50 people for a day and a half each month – Strategic Health Authority (SHA) Chief Executives, National Clinical Directors, Departmental Directors and others – as the *Top Team*. Its role was to review performance, agree next steps and provide leadership to the NHS. In the following days each of the SHA Chief Executives would hold a similar meeting with Trust and PCT Chief Executives and their own most senior people. In this way I and my colleagues centrally could send and receive messages to and from more than 1200 senior people very rapidly. They in turn discussed the issues with their Boards and senior teams.

The members of the Top Team were very senior and substantial figures in their own right. Each of the SHA Chief Executives for example were responsible for providing services for leading a system, that provided services to up to 3 million people with up to 50,000 staff and budgets up to £3 billion a year. Together they were a powerful group.

The Top Team provided a venue for shared performance review with SHA Chief Executives able to compare their local performance with others and challenge the laggards and be challenged in their turn. The meetings weren't just for sharing information and a chat. They could be very tough meetings with a lot of challenge of me and colleagues as well as of everybody else. I ran the meetings so that the SHAs and the national people all got equal time – this wasn't just a top down briefing session but at its best was a way of resolving problems and seeking and sharing solutions.

It was very important that we used this time together effectively so as to get results. Kate Barnard, who worked closely with me as Director of Development, helped us to agree the values and simple rules of engagement which are reproduced in Box 9.1.

I suspect that anyone who has participated in a Board or meeting will recognise the importance of "*honest closure*" and of making sure "*we speak well of each other – inside and outside meetings*". The list was born from our experience and recognised our different perspectives so that the last two about "*no surprises*" and early involvement were very much pleas from the SHA Chief Executives for those of us working at the centre to keep them engaged as new policies developed.

Box 9.1 The Top Team's Values and Simple Rules

Values

The work of the Team should be based on the following values:

- To lead not blame
- To work together not undermine each other
- To look for answers not give excuses
- To put the patient and public at the centre of our work.

Simple Rules

- When we collectively give authority to team members to act, we let them deliver
- We aim for agreement wherever possible and stick to it
- We aim for honest closure where we cannot agree
- We speak well of each other – inside and outside meetings
- We will try our hardest to work on a "no surprises" basis
- We involve each other as early as possible.

I also personally wrote a monthly Chief Executive's bulletin which dealt with core matters of information but also contained any messages I wanted to get across. I usually said something about the places I had visited in the last month or important events or meetings. Looking back on it now looks as much like a proto-blog as a bulletin. I deliberately made it very personal even though I sent it to about 2,000 people every month including all Chairs and Chief Executives in the NHS, Local Authority Chief Executives and Social Services Directors and anyone else who asked for it.

I saw the Bulletin as part of building relationships and committed myself to responding to anyone who wrote to me about something in it. This often led to very useful dialogue. I also told all Chief Executives in the NHS that they could telephone me at any time about any subject. A few did but no one abused the offer. The quid pro quo was that I would feel free to telephone them at any time – and did, sometimes to find out what was going on but sometimes also to offer support or congratulate them on some achievement.

This was all part of what I saw as building a *community of Chief Executives* and creating some form of collective leadership in order to develop greater solidarity and strength across the country. I held regular meetings in different parts of the country and annual Chief Executives' conferences as well as similar events for Chairs. Latterly, I also created a National Leadership Network for health and social care to bring together a wider group of leaders and continue the development of shared purpose.

There were many other management processes that, for example, assured formal accountability, monitored results and agreed business plans. We were very tough indeed on performance. I have chosen to emphasis this building of collective leadership here, as I did at the time, because I believe it was essential in holding the NHS together through a period of enormous change. Over these years the NHS was subject to a number of counter-cultural shocks – star ratings, re-organisations, the involvement of the private sector – all of them risked breaking the organisation apart. Moreover, the enthusiasm and good will that marked the start of the NHS Plan in 2000 had long since disappeared and there was considerable mistrust between many NHS leaders and the politicians.

This was obviously a very personal approach and one that tested my stamina and resilience. By far my greatest support came from my wife and family who put up with my absences and preoccupations and kept me grounded and sane. I was also supported by good colleagues and received excellent guidance both from Kate Barnard and from an external coach, Penny Jones. In general people aren't honest with Chief Executives. They either tell you what they think you want to hear or simply complain and criticise. On my visits around the NHS I had to give space first for people to voice their concerns before trying to get into a more honest and real dialogue.

Kate and Penny provided me with feedback, often gathered from others, and helped me to improve my own personal performance. How senior leaders behave, how they present themselves and their ideas and how they communicate are all very important. Influence, persuasion and leadership are all skills that coaching can improve.

There are many different ways of leading and managing organisations I suspect this sort of inclusive approach has wide application in healthcare systems with all their many stakeholders and leaders. Working together they can be very powerful, working against each other produces stalemate.

The build up of pressure

I have described in the last few chapters how pressure built up in the system. We were making a large number of changes at the same time, with new staff contracts and IT systems, increasing competition and the continuing struggle to reach demanding targets. Some of our policies, as we have seen, cut across each other. Decentralisation for example, made it more difficult to drive the IT programme from the centre in the way that might have been ideal.

I don't want to underestimate how difficult this was for some people in the NHS. Others, however, were able to gain some synergy from the different changes and use the process of becoming a Foundation Trust, for example, as a lever to implement contract changes, introduce new IT systems and improve both competitiveness and performance.

As Chief Executive I worked with the Top Team to try to make implementation as smooth and as well paced as possible. These major changes might perhaps have been implemented better if we had done them slower or one at a time; although we would have lost potential synergy and cumulatively they would have then taken us a decade or more. I wanted to get as much done as possible, however, and knew both that the big funding injection was due to run out in 2008 and suspected that the political will that had driven so much change would also weaken.

These questions of pace and timing aren't optional for a Chief Executive and senior team. They had to be answered. For good or ill we kept up the pace and, in what proved to be a mistake, I initiated a reorganisation of community services in July 2005. The intention was to separate PCTs from the management of community services so that they were better able to commission services without any potential conflict of interest. It was designed to create a better market place and allow for new organisations and more creative arrangements to be brought in.

These were sensible enough changes and implemented later. However, at the time the ground wasn't fully prepared, the proposals weren't as well thought through as they should have been and I hadn't got the new Secretary of State, Patricia Hewitt, fully engaged. A year earlier the old guiding coalition would have worked through and approved the plans. Now, I and colleagues had to liaise with new and inexperienced people without any background of shared experience and accumulated trust.

In retrospect I should have realised how much the environment had changed. Unfortunately, I didn't. It was complicated by the fact that the finances were getting out of control. As we saw in the last chapter, the rush for delivery, the expansion of facilities and staffing and competition were all pointing towards an overspend at the end of the year.

The real problem for me wasn't political or financial, however. It was more serious. I had chosen to base my authority and leadership on working closely with colleagues in the NHS and this reorganisation seriously damaged this crucial relationship. I had lost power and leverage. The environment had moved against me and, whilst nobody – other than one friend – told me I should go; I concluded that after 5 ½ years it was time to do so and retired the following spring.

I had done as much as I could as Chief Executive.

It was a sad moment but the timing was right for the NHS and probably for me. The NHS recovered under new leadership. The policies from that early period of reform carried on with continued improved performance and a new emphasis on quality.

The Prime Minister asked me to look at what more the UK could do with its experience and expertise to support improvement in developing countries. In doing so I discovered not just how much we could do but also how much we had to learn.[5]

Conclusions and key points

1. There are many leaders, informal and formal, in the NHS: clinical, managerial and non executive. Clinical leaders in particular have a very difficult but important role and can achieve things that others can't. However, the most important characteristic is the ability to work with others in teams across all the different divides.

2. Financial incentives can change behaviour but rarely motivate – and can demotivate by making people feel demeaned and cheapened. People in the NHS are motivated by many things including making a difference, being the best they can, feedback from patients and altruism.

3. Boards and governance generally have improved but need further development and will face further challenges. They potentially have a wider role to play in a more decentralised and locally focused NHS in the future.

4. Politicians have a major role to play in providing the will and the impetus for change, challenging the status quo and maintaining focus and momentum. However, they can also bring unhelpful ideological commitments to healthcare, excessively "spin" achievements, interfere inappropriately in operational issues and attract political attacks on the service itself.

Conclusions and key points (*Continued*)

5. The most successful period of reform was when there was a small group of politicians, managers and clinicians – a "guiding coalition" – at the top of the NHS who had established a way of working and communicating and were well aligned.

6. Nevertheless, despite the enthusiasm at the launch of the NHS Plan in 2000, tension and mistrust had developed between NHS leaders more widely and the politicians.

7. As Chief Executive I focused on results and inclusiveness, aiming to bring as many people and interests as possible into leadership roles which would help both hold the NHS together and create shared purpose and commitment. The Top Team played an important role in this. I also made sure that I understood and knew the NHS thoroughly, basing a large part of my authority and credibility on this.

References

1. Department of Health (2005) *A patient led NHS: delivering the NHS Improvement Plan;* 17 March, para 5.32, p. 33.
2. Emma Stanton and Claire Lemer (2010) *MBA for Medics*, Radcliffe.
3. Lords Hansard: 7 Dec 2007 column 1264.
4. Nigel Crisp (2009) The Department and the NHS – time for separation or a new relationship. *BMJ* **339**: 4881.
5. Nigel Crisp (2007) *Global Health Partnerships – the UK's contribution to health in developing countries.* TSO January.

Chapter 10

Patients, health and society

Late last year a friend of mine died from bowel cancer.

Tragically, Richard's cancer was discovered very late and at a stage when it had already spread so far that it was inoperable. His local NHS hospital provided him with chemotherapy – with all its attendant discomforts and side effects – but which also, very sadly, had little effect on the cancer which kept growing. At this point, thanks only to discussions with other patients, he became aware that there was a relatively new treatment available which might work but which he could only get privately.

He turned to the private sector. His new Consultant gave him a genetic test to see whether the new treatment was likely to work for him and, finding it did, put Richard on it. The results began to look good with the tumour reducing rapidly in the first few months. However, he immediately ran into problems with the insurers. Richard had medical insurance but at first the insurance company refused to cover his treatment. He won that argument but later, when he had already started the treatment – and it was showing hopeful signs of working – the company told him that they would only pay for it for a fixed period. After that time, at their discretion, the company would decide whether to continue funding or not.

Richard was outraged. As a lawyer with an eye for detail and contracts he began to unpick their arguments and, in doing so, to expose the way the whole insurance industry worked. He was one of the most determined people I have ever known and got his MP and me involved. Together we met representatives of the insurance company and, due to a comprehensive and thorough briefing from Richard, won that argument too. The company provided a list of other treatments that they would offer if his new treatment failed in the longer term. It was a very satisfactory outcome but Richard wasn't satisfied.

His investigations had shown him that there were a lot of other patients in a similar situation. Many of the people he met in the private clinic were in dispute with their insurers over what exactly they were covered for. Some had given up and were paying for themselves whilst others had given up the treatment. Richard turned to look at how this industry was regulated and found what he described as a mess with nobody in charge. Individual complaints are dealt with by one body, financial regulation by another, whilst the industry's own body seemed powerless to intervene when companies didn't live up to their Statement of Best Practice.

By this time I had talked to a number of Consultants and discovered that there is a great deal of unease about the way health insurers work and many tales of problems which affect both patients and clinicians. Several told me how much time they had to spend with insurers arguing about whether particular treatments are covered. Like Richard they told me that some insurers were much better than others. I also discovered, disturbingly, that very few clinicians were willing to speak about this on the record because they didn't want the insurers to discriminate against them or stop paying their fees.

This is all a far cry from the comforting adverts we have all seen from private health insurers with their reassurance that they will look after you. It seems very reminiscent of the US where decisions about treatment are taken by insurers in private and patients spend a great deal of time arguing their case.

Richard was let down both by the NHS and the private insurance sector. The NHS hadn't offered him screening so the tumour grew without any symptoms and without him knowing anything about it until it was too late. The NHS didn't offer him the new and more hopeful treatment he could get privately; although it is now available on the NHS. The private sector seemed to offer so much but gave him such problems with his insurance cover that it would have defeated a less determined person.

Richard's experience presents a shocking vision of the future – an NHS with crucial gaps, a private insurance sector which promises so much but fails to deliver and inadequate regulation.

We need to find ways to avoid it.

Patients and the public

Overall, patient satisfaction with the NHS grew during the NHS Plan years and public satisfaction nearly doubled between 1999 and 2009.[1] There remain, however, enormous issues to address which I divide here for convenience into three groups.

Firstly, as Richard's example shows there are gaps in screening and service provision which the NHS needs to address.

Secondly, some sectors of the population are served better than others and there are wide inequalities in access to healthcare and wide variations in the health and longevity of the population. The linkage between social issues and health is now well documented; with life expectancy in the poorest parts of the UK 10 years less than that in the most affluent.[2]

Thirdly, and underpinning the others, there is the need to understand better the perceptions, needs and wants of individuals and groups of patients and to shape services and the relationship between patients, staff and the NHS accordingly. This is the most complex area. Individual patients with the same condition and even from the same background may have very different needs from each other.

Moreover, some whole sectors of the population feel less well served than others. Patient and staff surveys regularly show, for example, that patients from black and minority ethnic communities are less satisfied with the NHS than those from the majority community and that staff from these communities similarly are less satisfied in their work.[3, 4]

This chapter starts by describing what we tried to do as part of the NHS Plan and in subsequent policies both to fill the service gaps and to deliver "*a health service designed around the patient*".[5] It continues by looking at some of the key issues about the engagement of patients and supporting them to take back control of their health and treatment. It follows this by addressing the issues of scrutiny – and holding the NHS to account – and questions how and why this has failed in the past. It builds on these discussions to consider how best to provide more patient centred services.

I have brought together here the issues of public health with those of individual patient care and autonomy in order to draw out the links between them. The chapter concludes by looking at the connections between health and society.

The NHS Plan and the waiting list dividend

The first years of implementation were very much focused on waiting lists, staff recruitment and service delivery. It was about dealing with some of the most high profile problems and filling some of the service gaps. Services improved for patients and there was some evidence of improved responsiveness to patients as competition and choice took hold. Essentially, however, this was about treating patients as consumers and as the recipients of services from others. Patients and citizens have other roles as well.

We needed these early results to gain some credibility and to buy time to deal with some of the issues like health promotion and patient engagement which would have the biggest long term impact but which would only show results slowly. We called it "the waiting list dividend" – bringing waiting lists down bought us the space to deal with these lower profile but perhaps more important issues.

Getting the timing right is vital. In Wales the administration had decided to focus first on public health issues and on building a strong health and local government infrastructure. It was an understandable and logical policy but the timing was wrong. As English waiting lists fell there was public pressure for them to change direction and start to deal with their own waiting lists before being able to return to the longer term issues. Scotland and Northern Ireland, too, had to respond to our progress.

We used the space created by the waiting list dividend to set out three important new policies from 2004 onwards. The first was a white paper – *Choosing Health: Making healthy choices easier* – published in November that year that attempted to set a new balance between the public's responsibilities and the state's.[6]

It was an important agenda. The Government had done a lot to try to tackle inequality and health – as opposed to healthcare issues – with greater funding transferred to poorer areas and setting Public Service Agreement targets for reducing smoking, improving health most quickly amongst the lower socio-economic groups 4 and 5 and improving outcomes for another disadvantaged group, children in care. It had also made sure that wider policies such as the Coronary Heart Disease NSF and Cancer Plan had a strong emphasis on health promotion – with a 5 a day fruit and vegetable campaign, free fruit in schools and *healthy schools* initiatives all linked to them. Elsewhere in government the *Sure Start* and nursery programmes were about giving children a healthy and positive start in life.

The white paper took these approaches further with proposed changes in legislation and regulation and led to cross departmental targets on obesity – where sport, education and health all had interests – and a great deal of encouragement for people to adopt healthy life styles.

The following March a social care green paper was published. *Independence, Well-being and Choice: Our Vision for the Future of Social Care for Adults in England* took a broadly similar perspective towards valuing the role of individuals, promoting what they could do for themselves as well as what Local Authorities could do for them.[7] A central theme was about enabling people to take control of their lives and to be as independent as possible.

This was supported by proposing greater use of individual budgets – an approach in which people with disabilities were able to receive the budget for their own care and spend it as they saw fit. Disability groups had long campaigned for this, arguing that they needed to control their own resources and gain independence to live the lives they wanted to live.

Both the earlier policy papers were followed up with a white paper, *Our health, our care, our say: a new direction for community services,*[8] in January 2006. It was based on extensive consultation with people throughout the country – through "town hall" meetings, individual interviews, focus groups and the like – about what they thought was needed for the future. Following this consultation, the white paper set out the principles which would underpin community services in the future with new types of services, greater engagement and participation of patients and much better information and support available for health promotion and disease prevention. It proposed extending individual budgets to wider groups of people.

These three policy documents were very consistent in content and approach and, whilst efforts were made to find ways to implement them, they essentially lacked teeth. By this stage national policies were very concentrated on decentralisation and local decision making so it wasn't possible to introduce many new national targets or earmark money for implementation. The inspectors in Social Care and Health could and did exercise some control. The few new cross-departmental targets – on obesity for example – were not perceived as central issues by many NHS leaders. They weren't the ones which were described earlier as "*targets you would get sacked for missing*" and they didn't have money attached.

The result of all this policy making and consultation was to widen awareness of the issues and build a foundation of knowledge and models for the future. There was relatively little impact in the short term. Mainstream thinking had shifted a bit perhaps, but power hadn't.

There were, however, three very significant legacies of these few years. The first which the Chief Medical Officer, Sir Liam Donaldson and other doctors had campaigned for years was a ban on smoking in public places, including pubs, restaurants, and clubs. It was implemented very smoothly and will have long term dividends. Liam described it as "*probably the most significant achievement since the devastating consequences of smoking for public health were established beyond doubt.*"[9]

The second was the development of policies for individual budgets which seem to offer great promise for the future by recognising the roles that are best played by the individual and the authority and can offer holistic health and social care.

The third, closely linked to this, was the development of ideas and programmes for promoting all aspects of patient involvement, engagement and control.

The involvement of patients is not just a superficial or desirable add-on. There is plenty of evidence that patient involvement in their own care and a good experience of care are associated with better clinical outcomes.[10] We also know that the greatest health need and the greatest cost to the NHS now comes from people with long term conditions, often elderly and often with more than one infirmity. Moreover, the greatest risks to health now come from life style related issues – only individuals can decide whether or not to change the way they live. This has to be a priority for the NHS.

Engagement, participation and patient control

The NHS Plan described a "*service designed around the patient*". Soon after it was published the patients groups on the Modernisation Board began to point out that this was old fashioned and rather patronising wording and that "*around the patient*" should be changed to "*with the patient*" if not to something more empowering that recognised the primacy of patients and their role as much more than passive consumers.

Harry Cayton, who had been Chief Executive of the Alzheimer's Society for 12 years and a member of the Modernisation Board, became the Department's first

Director for Patients and the Public in 2003. He accelerated this thinking and brought fresh insight into the top of the NHS and the Department.

Three big themes stand out from that period. The first, the *Expert Patient Programme*, was based on the idea that patients with long term conditions were not only the experts on their particular manifestation of the disease but knew more about it in general than clinicians. They therefore needed to be given the space and any training they needed to manage their own condition. They could also support other patients, particularly those newly diagnosed; take a lead role in designing more appropriate services; and help train clinicians and carers.

It is a very powerful idea which had been developed in the UK primarily by a voluntary group, Arthritis Care, and based on a programme at Stanford University. In an interesting series of developments the department took the idea up, re-named it the *Expert Patient Programme*, widened its scope and sought to spread it through the NHS. We were still routinely earmarking funds at the time and gave each PCT £5,000 to develop a local scheme. It was one of the more successful of such initiatives and many schemes developed around the country.

In an interesting final twist the Department recognised that having incubated the idea and fostered its development, the Programme would be able to develop its potential still further as an independent entity. It therefore spun off the programme as the first national Community Interest Company – a relatively new structure which allows a body to trade and operate as a business but with a social purpose – in 2006. It thrives today as the Expert Patient Programme CIC.

Harry also led the development of wider policies of shared care and co-production. He coined the idea of the *"flat pack patient"* – the patient who was able to get all the constituent parts for his or her care from the health system but then assembled it him or herself, possibly but not necessarily with help from the professional.[11] The point was that in reality many patient consultations work best when they bring together the clinical wisdom and knowledge of the professional and the practical wisdom and experience of the patients. The patient and the professional are co-workers.

In the words of Al Mulley, a Harvard Professor who has done a lot of research on shared decision making, *"Every patient brings their own context"*.[12] Each patient has their own particular view of themselves and the world where their own experience, culture, knowledge and spirituality guide their conscious or unconscious responses to the professional and the proposed treatment. Shared care and shared decision making are about finding the best ways to meld and match the skills and experience of both and in Al Mulley's words for the professional to *"confer agency on the patient"* by putting his or her skills and knowledge at the patient's disposal.

The Wanless Review which provided some of the intellectual underpinning for the big boost in NHS expenditure talked about patient engagement as key to the future of the NHS.[13] Even this rather misses some of the subtleties here. It is not so much about the professionals engaging, or as it is sometimes put, empowering patients; but about stopping disengaging them and stopping disempowering them. In reality it is patients who most often engage the professionals by going to them for help and empowering them to do things on our behalf.

Patients make many of the decisions in healthcare consciously or by default. We need only look at how many medications are not used as prescribed, how much treatment is abandoned part way through and how many vaccinations are refused – let alone how many of us go on drinking, eating and doing other health threatening things despite the best evidence and the best advice. Patients only reliably do what the professional tells them when they are feeling very ill or in great danger. As they feel better they are more and more likely to make their own decision and their own trade-offs about whether to follow the clinician's advice or instructions.[14]

Other examples show us that even with potentially life threatening conditions like cancer and stroke there is an enormous variation in whether or not people seek treatment on the basis of their early symptoms – and often this depends on the influence of friends and family members.[15, 16] This isn't about what people say they do or how they behave towards professionals, when they are still often very deferential. It is about what they actually do in reality: a sort of passive resistance not an active one or just a polite independence. The only way for professionals to handle this is to find ways to get fully alongside their patients.[17]

The implication of this way of thinking is that the NHS needs to enable patients to have as much knowledge and control as possible. This takes us into the third area: the provision of health coaches and the creation of what have now become Personal Health Budgets. A number of programmes have developed locally around the NHS where health coaches are available to individuals and groups with particular risks factors; whilst peer counsellors have been use in many neighbourhoods and communities. Even more recently, and after the period covered by this book, new ideas have been developed about how to market healthy behaviour to groups and individuals and about how social networks can encourage or discourage such behaviour. Put simply – and as we all know – we are very heavily influenced by our peers and by the company we keep.

The policy of personal health budgets has also developed but not yet as far as it might. Harry Cayton wants to take patient-led healthcare much further. He has written about the *patient entrepreneur* who is able to take charge of their own health and influence and shape what healthcare providers do.[18] In a recent conversation he told me that "*we got very near to enabling patients to have some really autonomy with personal budgets but we stepped back from the brink – we were afraid of losing control and about what they would do with it*". Perhaps next time we won't be.

The NHS works hard to reduce the burden of disease for patients and populations. Sadly, we know that treatment – from course of chemotherapy to weekly visits to a surgery for blood tests – also imposes a burden. Maureen Bisognano, the President of the Institute for Healthcare Improvement, has called for health systems to work at reducing the burden of treatment as well as the burden of disease.[19] In the same speech she talked about the importance of helping patients develop resilience in the face of adversity.

These very human issues are often picked up very effectively by patients groups and voluntary organisations which create solidarity and provide support for individuals as well as acting as experts and advocating for improvement.

Patient voice and scrutiny

Patients and patients' groups have other roles, too, as watchdog organisations or as individual citizens in holding the NHS to account and querying its decisions. The NHS has never been very successful in finding the right balance in either aspect.

Community Health Councils were created in every Health Authority area in 1974 with the triple roles of supporting individual patients with complaints, monitoring local services and engaging in consultation on proposed service changes. They had a chequered history with some becoming overtly political and some, at the other extreme, so much influenced by the local NHS as to be useless. They were abolished in the NHS Plan and their functions split apart.

Patient Advocacy and Liaison Services (PALS) were created within each Trust to support individuals with their concerns and complaints and to offer information. Patients Forums were also established in each Trust to feed in views and perceptions and advise on services. Local Authorities were given the power of scrutiny of NHS plans locally and the health and social care inspectors maintained their roles. The three new bodies and processes were supplemented with better public access to information, a new right of redress and arrangements for patient involvement in all NHS bodies. These new arrangements have only had partial success.

There are some good examples, of course. Some of the PALS have been very effective in supporting individuals. The governance arrangements for Foundation Trusts which include local elections and patient governors have worked well in some cases. Local Government scrutiny of plans has in some places helped build good local relationships and planning arrangements. CHI and its successors as inspectors have picked up problems and instituted inquiries. NICE and other bodies have very good means of involving patients and members of the public in decision making.

However, none of these things stopped the long delay in tackling MRSA or the scandal at the Mid Staffordshire NHS Foundation Trust. The final Report of the Mid Staffordshire NHS Foundation Trust Inquiry into events between January 2005 and March 2009 makes devastating reading.[20] It describes appalling treatment and neglect of patients. Witnesses tell of soiled sheets left unchanged, patients left on bed pans for an hour, buzzers unanswered, staff who were present refusing to give help, high levels of falls, unsupervised patients suffering from dementia, poor hygiene and much more.

The Report says that "*The culture of the Trust was not conducive to providing good care for patients or providing a supportive working environment for staff*" and goes on to list 10 contributory factors – attitudes of patients and staff, bullying, target-driven priorities, disengagement from management, low staff morale, isolation, lack of openness, acceptance of poor standards of conduct, reliance on external assessments and denial.[21]

It is a tragic local failure but we are all implicated. The problems went on for a long time without being brought into the open. All the governance and inspection systems appear to have failed. Two points about patients stand out. The Report says that *patients' attitudes were characterised by a reluctance to insist on receiving basic care or medication for fear of upsetting staff.*"[22] The second was that a patients' group knew about the problems and was campaigning for a long time before anyone responded.

Mid Staffordshire illustrates the tensions in the NHS's mixed management and regulation system and begs the question of how the current system of local control and national policy and regulation can ensure that such a scandal never happens again. It also illustrates two fundamental points about patient and public involvement. The first is the imbalance in power between the professionals and the patients – patients were afraid of upsetting staff. The second is how to give patients' groups legitimacy and clout. Neither can be solved easily.

I won't comment further on Mid Staffordshire because a Public Inquiry is underway and will report this year. Other Inquiries, like the 3 medical ones I described in Chapter 2, have made recommendations that have improved the NHS. No doubt this one will too.

It is much more than patient and public scrutiny that is needed, however. Boards, patient Governors and senior managers need to have very good ways of staying in touch with what is happening at the front line. It is not just about walkabouts, important as they are in gauging culture. This isn't enough. Boards need a systematic way of being alerted to issues, helping them to identify the precise problem and deciding how to deal with it.

Health and society

Patients and staff issues often interlink. Unhappy and stressed staff won't give their best. Morale affects patient care, as seen in Mid Staffordshire. Both patient and staff issues are also linked to wider social ones.

This chapter has concentrated on people as patients of the NHS but has continually touched on links with the wider community and, in particular, with social services. Healthcare and social care is a combination that many adults, particularly elderly ones, require in order to live active lives. It is not the only combination. Children need education and healthcare. Families may need financial support, help in gaining employment and very often housing. High crime levels link with poor health, violence, insecurity, drug and solvent abuse, poverty and mental illness. All these connections are known and documented yet health is often treated as a subject apart, kept within its hierarchies and organisations.

There were several attempts to shift the boundaries and create better working arrangements between different organisations throughout these years. There were many successes with effective Drug Action Teams, Community Mental Health Teams and outreach and intermediate care services designed to provide care at home and keep people out of hospital.

Staff on these teams often had to work against their own systems to make the service work effectively – respecting, for example, the different confidentiality rules and rights of access to data and the different levels of accountability different staff members could hold – but still making sure enough information was shared to provide the treatment and care necessary. Budgetary processes, planning cycles, IT systems and staff term and conditions all had to be worked round. Most of these partnerships and programmes worked because people made them do so. They built the relationships and took the risks they needed to in order to be successful. They were entrepreneurial.

This is a crucial area for the future. Despite all these difficulties, the support many patients and service users need will only come through joint working across all these barriers and from bringing patients and service users into the collaboration.

Health is integrated in reality, if not organisationally, into every level of public service in a community. It also influences and is influenced by wider social issues. Let me take as an example a point I made at the beginning of the chapter about patients and staff from black and minority ethnic communities being less happy with the NHS than the majority of the population. There are moral and legal issues here but there is also a very significant health one. The NHS was not serving a significant part of its population as well as it should.

I decided to make this a leadership issue for Chief Executives and Chairs and with help from Kate Barnard and a group of people from black and minority ethnic groups drew up and published a Leadership Race Equality Plan in February 2004.[23] It contained five points about health services and five about developing people. These included making sure that all planning documents addressed race equality, that there was monitoring in place and training and development opportunities available. I also decided to make it personal.

The problems were both personal and institutional. They were about how people perceived the way they were treated, but also about what the evidence showed. Some communities have particularly needs, with people from a South Asian background, for example, being much more susceptible to diabetes and heart disease than others. There were questions to consider about how well such services were aligned with cultural and behavioural norms and questions, too, about why young black men were many times more likely to be in mental hospitals than their white peers.

At that time there were about 7% of the national population from these black and minority ethnic communities but they made up 17% of NHS staff. How they were treated by the NHS was also therefore of importance in how people felt about their country as a whole. Analysis showed that people were clustered in the lower paid parts of the organisation with very few Directors and Chief Executives. The NHS was "snow capped"; it became whiter – and my black friends said chillier – the higher up the organisation you went. Looking from below it didn't look as if black people were welcome as leaders in the NHS.

This was important as a health issue because we needed to have talented people from any and every background able to contribute to the full. It was also important that we had senior people who understood the different issues facing different communities and whose presence at the top would give those communities confidence that their concerns would be heard.

I focussed the Plan on senior leaders in the NHS and said, without setting an actual target, that I hoped by July that 500 of them would be mentoring a member of staff from an ethnic minority. In the event 900 were doing so by that date. I think that for most of the white NHS leaders this was really a co-mentoring process.

The first person I mentored, Yvonne Coghill, was black, a woman, a nurse and worked in the community. I was none of those things and learned a great deal from her perspective on the NHS. I was able to see how national policies impacted in her world and how people at her level in the organisation and from her background reacted to the changes we were making. For her part she gained insight into a very different world and learned how decisions were made and how people behaved at the top of the organisation. I don't know which of us learned more.

Yvonne is now leading the very successful *Breaking Through Initiative* which supports people from black and ethnic minority communities to develop and progress through the organisation. The graduates from Breaking Through are now starting to appear in senior roles around the organisation.

The mentoring experience reinforced my understanding of the importance of relationships in the NHS. Systems and structures are helpful but relationships – being able to work with and draw the best from others – are essential. Many senior leaders told me how transforming the mentoring experience had been for them. It gave perspective, background and depth to their understanding of the people they were working with as colleagues and serving as patients. The sad truth at the time, as I recall from a newspaper article, was that only about 10% of white people over the age of 50 had a black friend. Many of us were around 50.

There are other excluded groups including young white working class men. A GP friend reminded me that middle class NHS leaders also have few friends in this group and may have difficulty in seeing the world as they do. Leaders need to find good ways of connecting more widely, and leadership positions need to be opened up to everyone.

Race, ethnicity and cultural issues are as important in the NHS as they are in any part of our society. The NHS can work at its best when it is part of a community wide effort and part of a healthy society. It can contribute to this and gain from it.

Health and power

This chapter has identified some of the best new thinking and practice in the NHS but has also described some of the worst. It opened with an account of how both the NHS and private insurance failed my friend Richard. It is very difficult to make sense of it all and to understand why there are these wide variations and what, if anything, can be done about them.

There are common themes here about who exercises power and makes decisions about individuals and services, about the importance of relationships as opposed to structures and processes and about people – patients and members of staff – being entrepreneurial.

It is worth noting here, however, how crucial this linkage is between health and wider social issues and between the NHS and other local service structures and organisations. One of the themes of the whole book is to understand better how we might move from a hospital and professional based service to a more community and people based one. There are many powerful interests which support the continuance of the old model. Patients' groups and local institutions and services could, if they found a way of making themselves more aligned with each other, begin to build a countervailing power and help achieve change.

In order to do so they need to create a new shared vision for the NHS.

Wider aims for the NHS

This discussion about the NHS and society suggests that it has a wider role in the community than is sometimes evident or recognised. I believe it needs to make this more explicit in the future and change the way it works accordingly. As I will argue in Chapter 12, the NHS needs to contribute to the wider goal of helping people to live a life they have reason to value, as part of a healthy society and a healthy world.

Conclusions and key points

1. There are gaps in NHS provision which need to be addressed. Private insurance with its financial limits and private decision making is no substitute.

2. Improving waiting times and other high profile problem areas gave us the "waiting list dividend" – the space and time to focus on longer term issues such as health promotion and patient engagement which will have the greatest long term benefits.

3. Despite the development of good and consistent policy statements on health, social care and community services there were relatively few achievements – with the very notable exception of the ban on smoking in public places – because implementation plans lacked teeth.

4. There was a great deal of creative thinking about engaging patients and enabling them to exercise more control in partnership with professionals – including the development of personal health budgets, the expert patient programme, the use of health coaches and the promotion of patients as entrepreneurs.

5. New arrangements were put in place for external scrutiny and oversight of the NHS but they and the internal governance arrangements failed in Mid Staffordshire. They need revision.

6. Health and social issues are intimately linked. Local services need to be developed and run in partnership with each other, despite the many barriers to doing so.

7. Power needs to be redistributed in the NHS in order to move from a hospital and doctor based system to a community and person based one. Patient's groups and local institutions and services could, if they found a way of aligning themselves, begin to create a counterbalance to powerful interests invested in the status quo.

References

1. National Centre for Social Research (2011) *SN 6695 – British Social Attitudes Survey* 2009, Feb.
2. World Health Organisation (2008) *Closing the gap in a generation: Health equity through action on the social determinants of health*; Commission on Social Determinants of Health.

3. Office for National Statistics (2008) *Report on self reported experience of patients from black and minority ethnic groups*, May.

4. Campbell JL, Ramsay J, Green J. (2001) Age, gender, socioeconomic, and ethnic differences in patients' assessments of primary health care. *Qual Health Care* **10**: 90–5.

5. Department of Health (2000) *The NHS Plan: a plan for investment, a plan for reform;* CM4818–I, July, p. 17.

6. Department of Health (2004) *Choosing Health: Making healthy choices easier;* Cm 6364, 16 Nov.

7. Department of Health (2005) *Independence, Well-being and Choice: Our Vision for the Future of Social Care for Adults in England;* CM 6499, 21st March.

8. Department of Health (2006) *Our health, our care, our say: a new direction for community services;* CM 6737 31st Jan.

9. Department of Health (2010) *Advancing Health – examples of the work of Chief Medical Officer for England, 1998–2010;* 14 March.

10. Fremont AM, Clearly PD, Hargraves JL, Rowe RM, Jacobsen NB, Ayanian JZ (2001) Patient-centered processes of care and long-term outcomes of acute myocardial infarction. *J Gen Int Med* **14**: 800–8.

11. Harry Cayton (2008) The flat-pack patient? Creating health together, *Patient Education and Counseling* **62**(3), Sept.

12. Mulley AG (2009) The need to confront variations in practice. *BMJ* **339**: 1007–9

13. Derek Wanless (2002) *Our future health: taking a long-term view;* HM Treasury, April.

14. Nigel Crisp (2010) *Turning the World Upside Down;* RSM Press, Jan, p 129ff.

15. Leydon GM, Bynoe-Sutherland J, Coleman MP (2003) The journey towards a cancer diagnosis: the experiences of people with cancer, their families and carers. *European Journal of Cancer Care* (English) **12**(4): 317–26.

16. Kiko L, Hupcey JE (2008) Factors that influence health-seeking behaviors of patients experiencing acute stroke. *Journal of Neuroscience Nursing*, **40**(6):333–40.

17. Katherine Hobson (2011) How can you help the medicine go down? *Wall Street Journal*, 28 March.

18. Cayton H (2007) Patients as entrepreneurs: Who is in charge of change? In: Anderson E, Tritter J and Wilson R: *Health Democracy – The future of involvement in health and social care;* NHS, The National Centre for Involvement.

19. Maureen Bisognano (2010) President's address to Institute of Healthcare National Forum, Florida, 7 Dec.

20. Mid Staffordshire NHS Foundation Trust Inquiry Final Report February 2010.

21. Ibid. paras 14 and 15.

22. Ibid. para 14.

23. Department of Health (2004) *The Leadership Race Equality Plan*, Electronic publication 13 Feb.

Chapter 11

Conclusions and key points

This chapter tries to answer the question I am constantly asked: *What can we learn from the English experience of reform and improvement?*

It brings together the conclusions and key issues from each chapter – with some minor editing to reduce duplication – and without the stories and the background explanations.

Readers may wish to study it, skim read it or skip it all together before going on to what I believe this history suggests would be reasonable strategies for the future in England, other countries and the global institutions which are described in the following three chapters.

Chapter 1: 24 hours to save the NHS

1. In 2000 there was real doubt as to whether the NHS could survive. It did so thanks to a major act of political will, radical reforms and massively increased funding. Public satisfaction almost doubled, patients returned from the private sector and a new political consensus about maintaining the NHS was established.

2. Action was centred on the NHS Plan which targeted improvements in priority areas including cutting waiting times for services dramatically, making it easier for people to get healthcare, reducing premature deaths from cancer and coronary heart disease, increasing staffing numbers and improving facilities.

3. There were four main areas of reform:
   a. Service redesign and improvement
   b. System reform
   c. Restructuring the workforce
   d. Knowledge, technology and science.

4. The design of the reforms was very important but implementation also required a relentless working through of the details; planning and adjusting plans as circumstances dictated.

5. The NHS may have been saved but it is not yet sustainable. There is once again a need for a radical approach which will enable the NHS to transition from a service focussed on hospitals, doctors and disease treatment to one

which is community based, people centred and geared towards prevention and promotion.

6. The NHS needs to develop a new approach that goes beyond managerialism and the medical model, keeping the best aspects of both, meeting people where they are and supporting them in how they want to live their lives.

7. There are many lessons here for the NHS in the future and for other countries both about the design of reforms and about implementation. The UK can also learn from other countries including those which don't have our resources or our baggage and our vested interests and are freer to innovate.

Chapter 2: The national and global context

1. By 1999 the NHS had multiple problems and was in decline. Poor systems, lack of resources, low morale and an absence of overall direction all contributed to inadequate clinical results and unsatisfactory care for patients.

2. The overall framework of the NHS with its emphasis on primary care and equity was robust. However, in order to survive the NHS needed a clear direction, greater unity of purpose, new energy and resources and a radical overhaul of systems, incentives and organisation. Incremental changes would not do. This required a massive reform programme and a major act of political will.

3. Health is always a political issue and the provision of healthcare is very closely related to how people see the world and what aspirations they have for their society. It can't be treated in isolation from other social and economic policies. Health reform in the UK was part of wider efforts to re-define and re-shape the 50 year old Welfare State.

4. There are many different perspectives in healthcare and many powerful interests. The strength of these provider and staff interests can serve patients and the public well but they can also distort priorities and lead to a closed and patronising culture which doesn't listen to patient's needs or value their views.

5. There have been three broad shifts in power over the years with doctors giving up some power to other groups, the professions becoming more closed and powerful, and the public becoming more demanding. These all shaped the reforms.

6. New ways are needed to promote patients and citizens as a counter balance to the power of the professions and other interests and to engage them more fully in their own care and in the design of services.

7. Four major global trends affect planning and policy:
   a. Non-communicable diseases and long term conditions are now the main causes or illness and death and the biggest consumers of healthcare resources. Community and people based services are needed for

these diseases to replace the hospital and doctor based services which were required 50 years ago.

b. Patients and the public are becoming both more assertive and more important in the prevention, cure and management of disease.

c. Technology and science are providing new solutions which require new services to be designed and make old ways of working redundant.

d. The world is becoming ever more interdependent in health terms with the global spread of diseases, reliance on the same resources and staff and the need to align policies regionally and globally.

8. The financial situation is likely to force the choice about whether the NHS restricts the services available or takes the harder option of changing the way it provides services and releases costs from the old infrastructure and traditional practices.

Chapter 3: The NHS Plan – overview of the story

1. The creation and launch of the NHS Plan was a very successful exercise in getting Prime Ministerial, cross Government and stakeholder support as well as funding for a major transformation programme.

2. The Plan set a clear direction and was very ambitious with more than 200 targets of different sorts – for inputs, service improvements and health outcomes. The number of targets and an inherent tension between a top down and a bottom up approach were to be problems in the years to come.

3. Mobilisation takes time and there was a significant lag of more than a year before results started to come through. This was both frustrating and problematic. The Government resorted to a series of small scale initiatives to maintain momentum during this period.

4. The NHS had to deal both with the day to day management of services as well as with more unusual events like Public Inquiries at the same time as introducing reforms. Success in managing "winter pressures" helped build confidence whilst waiting for results.

5. At the outset and in order to kick start change there needed to be very firm leadership and very clear accountability, particularly in an organisation like the NHS which was in practice very decentralised and had many different leaders.

6. Firm leadership and service re-design were not enough by themselves and more radical system reforms were introduced which took the NHS and many of the Government's natural supporters out of their comfort zone and caused a great deal of controversy.

7. The mixture of the four areas of reform – service re-design, system reform, staff restructuring and better use of knowledge, science and technology – complimented each other and accelerated change.

Chapter 4: Service improvement and delivery

1. There were enormous improvements in targeted areas. Maximum hospital waiting times fell by three quarters and the median by two thirds. Premature deaths from cancer, coronary heart disease and from suicide fell as planned. New services and new ways of accessing services became available to the public. Activity levels rose very fast as services expanded and improved.

2. Initially there were psychological and confidence barriers to overcome as well as inertia and some opposition. "Star ratings" gave an early shock to the system and helped start improvement.

3. A two part approach of firm performance management and accountability on the one hand and assistance with quality improvement on the other brought results. The innovation of quality improvement needed to be matched with the persistent and daily grind of delivery.

4. A simple model of improvement was developed which involved a clear target and measurement, clinical leadership, knowledge of best practice, local adaptation and clear accountability for delivery. It was applied to everything from reducing MRSA to preventing suicides and speeding up services.

5. At its best "the system learned" as the formal mechanisms of communication were aided by informal structures and networks in making improvement. We all learned together.

6. It was important to provide many ways for the public to access services both to improve health but also to secure public support and confidence.

7. As services improved more people used them and the use of the private sector declined – providing external validation of improvement.

8. Improvement could be accelerated by bringing in system reforms alongside the improvement and management processes.

Chapter 5: System reforms

1. Reform and re-design of the system can bring big benefits. However, these sorts of reforms – involving such radical changes as introducing private sector provision into a state system – are of intense public and political interest and can't be handled by clinicians and managers alone.

2. In the UK as we moved from essentially a nationalised industry approach to healthcare to a national health system which made use of other providers we came up against political, public and staff opposition. We were dealing with some issues which had helped define the NHS since its inception in 1948. It was about symbolism as well as practical reality.

3. Decentralisation brings benefits but needs to take place within a clear national framework and may require the initial strengthening of the centre so that subsequent decentralisation is coherent and effective. We planned to move from an 80:20 top down approach to a 20:80 bottom up one but recognised this would not be a smooth progression from one to the other.

4. Decentralisation shifts power from one group to another and will inevitably be opposed to some extent by the losers. It therefore needs to be led and implemented firmly. It also requires a new framework to secure quality and appropriate regulation.

5. Offering patients more choice made relatively little impact initially on their behaviour but it did affect the way NHS organisations reacted and thereby created some significant improvements. It also revealed some deep seated paternalistic and, even, protectionist attitudes amongst professionals and policy makers.

6. Whilst private sector providers were initially introduced into the NHS to create additional capacity they were retained to provide continued competition. However, the extent of their involvement was limited and they operated within the overall NHS framework.

7. All these changes had a cost. Expansion of the private sector meant reductions in NHS capacity and activity. These costs needed to be anticipated and actively managed. However, political considerations made it hard to do this with the result that problems were stored up for the future.

8. The radical nature and the number of changes tested both the unity of the NHS and the relationship between politicians and executives. It was very important to have good mechanisms – like the Top Team – for ensuring that the whole of the senior leadership were able to participate in decision making and be willing to buy in to the whole process and its consequences.

9. Improvement had to be maintained **and** it had to be publicised to ensure momentum and show that the NHS could improve and was improving.

Chapter 6: The NHS workforce

1. Restructuring of the workforce and re-design of jobs is essential to deal with changed circumstances and manage costs. Incentives can help but local leaders – in particular doctors – can make significant changes where external managers cannot. The GPs in particular led a great deal of change.

2. All the HR policies were linked to the *skills escalator* whereby an individual could progress up the organisation gaining experience, skills and reward on the way; whilst roles could be passed down the organisation as new systems and technology allowed and appropriate systems were put in place.

3. There were many problems recruiting staff at the beginning of the period but improved pay and terms of conditions as well as higher levels of education and training meant that target levels of increases in staffing were exceeded.

4. Wider policy issue such as the European Working Times Directive and changes in taxation affect health policy and costs.

5. The major programmes for changing pay and terms and conditions created streamlined and more flexible arrangements, but many benefits were not realised in the short term – and, in the GPs contract, led to large costs over runs.

6. The difficulties in implementation were largely due to: many things happening at once; a disconnect between the people negotiating and those implementing which was reinforced by increasing decentralisation; and Government playing too many roles from funder to negotiator and NHS champion. Some issues also became very politicised. Managers need to choose whether to make changes sequentially or concurrently – either way there will be problems that need to be managed.

7. Underlying all these issues is a wider problem of motivation. Making changes in pay and terms and conditions is very difficult and can de-motivate even when pay increases.

Chapter 7: Knowledge, science and technology

1. The National Programme for IT had many successes in improving patient care and costs – from digitised images to the secure NHS network and electronic prescribing – which put England amongst the world leaders in the field. The procurement process was robust and effective, changing Government policy and putting the NHS in a strong position with its suppliers. Costs were well controlled.

2. Problems mainly with the Care Records Service have, however, damaged the reputation of the whole Programme. These were due to design issues, over-centralisation and midstream changes in the implementation programme. These problems were compounded by politics, by difficulties in providing clinical leadership and lack of agreement amongst clinicians and by the range of other priorities facing NHS organisations.

3. The model of implementation used elsewhere on clinical issues like MRSA and waiting times didn't work where clinicians had no special knowledge. There are many lessons to learn from making large scale change involving thousands of people.

4. The NHS estate has been rejuvenated with more than 100 new hospital developments and 3000 refurbishments in primary care. New buildings and new designs are helping support the more diverse and flexible range of

services needed in the future. PFI has been crucial. Here as elsewhere the rush to achieve targets wasted some opportunities for redesign but over time new and better processes have been established.

5. The UK plays a leading role internationally in generating evidence and in knowledge management. NICE has a strengthened its role in providing evidence for patients as well as clinicians and policy makers. It is essential to have an independent organisation to identify evidence and knowledge, challenge common assumptions and sometimes reveal unpalatable truths.

6. Introducing innovation in healthcare is difficult for local reasons to do with the structure and culture of the NHS but is also influenced by the wider ways in which clinicians adapt and learn.

7. NHS leaders increasingly need to understand and integrate the contribution that these technical issues – IT, design and knowledge management – play in developing and delivering high quality services.

8. There has been very good progress in R and D in creating a focus on service issues and in developing the NHS as a learning laboratory. The Department, the NHS, academia, research institutes and industry have made progress in coming together to create a common platform for the benefit of patients and the UK.

9. There are policy issues to address about how much science and technology can focus on early health not late disease; provide access to all not just the few; and help create independence rather than dependence – and in so doing create global public goods, not purely private products for commercial exploitation.

Chapter 8: Finance and productivity

1. There always need to be priorities in health. Financial measures and *payment by results* can ensure they get attention; whilst financial allocations can be used to deliver funding to the poorest and least healthy populations in the country.

2. By 2006 the "rush for delivery", new facilities and staff becoming available and the pressures of competition led to a build up of financial pressure in the system and to the NHS overspending. The NHS returned to surplus the following year but is now facing severe financial difficulty with virtually no real term growth for the next four years.

3. The Private Finance Initiative was the major funder of hospital developments with over £12 billion invested and more committed to LIFT for community and primary care premises. After early problems, the NHS and its partners learned how to manage the process effectively and have delivered many fine new buildings. The PFI capital has to be paid for in annual instalments which

may eventually amount to 2 to 3% of annual spend. Similar levels of costs would have been incurred by any capital programme.

4. There are no generally agreed ways of assessing the productivity of a health system like the NHS and there are particular difficulties in accounting for prevention work and quality improvements. The best available measures which take some account of quality gains suggest that productivity shrank by about 1.5% a year in the early years as the new funding flowed in and that it improved to a neutral position as the results appeared thereafter. There appear to be some new and promising ways of measuring the actual value of health gained through particular interventions.

5. Despite the massive increases in the NHS budget UK health spending is still lower than almost all its main comparator countries. Many of them had similar levels of increased funding over this period, although none appears to have had the same planned investment as part of a development strategy.

6. The UK's performance improved relative to most other comparator countries during this period. The NHS in England, which alone implemented the NHS Plan, significantly outperformed the other UK countries during this period.

7. The independent Healthcare Commission identified "*some dramatic progress*" as well as areas like inequalities and obesity to concentrate on for the future.

Chapter 9: Leadership

1. There are many leaders, informal and formal, in the NHS: clinical, managerial and non executive. Clinical leaders in particular have a very difficult but important role and can achieve things that others can't. However, the most important characteristic is the ability to work with others in teams across all the different divides.

2. Financial incentives can change behaviour but rarely motivate – and can de-motivate by making people feel demeaned and cheapened. People in the NHS are motivated by many things including making a difference, being the best they can, feedback from patients and altruism.

3. Boards and governance generally have improved but need further development and will face further challenges. They potentially have a wider role to play in a more decentralised and locally focused NHS in the future.

4. Politicians have a major role to play in providing the will and the impetus for change, challenging the status quo and maintaining focus and momentum. However, they can also bring unhelpful ideological commitments to healthcare, excessively "spin" achievements, interfere inappropriately in operational issues and attract political attacks on the service itself.

5. The most successful period of reform was when there was a small group of politicians, managers and clinicians – a "guiding coalition" – at the top of the NHS who had established a way of working and communicating and were well aligned.

6. Nevertheless, despite the enthusiasm at the launch of the NHS Plan in 2000, tension and mistrust had developed between NHS leaders more widely and the politicians.

7. As Chief Executive I focused on results and inclusiveness, aiming to bring as many people and interests as possible into leadership roles which would help both hold the NHS together and create shared purpose and commitment. The Top Team played an important role in this. I also made sure that I understood and knew the NHS thoroughly, basing a large part of my authority and credibility on this.

Chapter 10: Patients, health and society

1. There are gaps in NHS provision which need to be addressed. Private insurance with its financial limits and private decision making is no substitute.

2. Improving waiting times and other high profile problem areas gave us the "waiting list dividend" – the space and time to focus on longer term issues such as health promotion and patient engagement which will have the greatest long term benefits.

3. Despite the development of good and consistent policy statements on health, social care and community services there were relatively few achievements – with the very notable exception of the ban on smoking in public places – because implementation plans lacked teeth.

4. There was a great deal of creative thinking about engaging patients and enabling them to exercise more control in partnership with professionals – including the development of personal health budgets, the expert patient programme, the use of health coaches and the promotion of patients as entrepreneurs.

5. New arrangements were put in place for external scrutiny and oversight of the NHS but they and the internal governance arrangements failed in Mid Staffordshire. They need revision.

6. Health and social issues are intimately linked. Local services need to be developed and run in partnership with each other, despite the many barriers to doing so.

7. Power needs to be redistributed in the NHS in order to move from a hospital and doctor based system to a community and person based one. Patient's groups and local institutions and services could, if they found a way of aligning themselves, begin to create a counterbalance to powerful interests invested in the status quo.

Chapter 12

The future of the NHS in England

It looks as if a political fix has been done to manage the current disagreements about policy on the NHS, but there is no quick fix for the long term challenges it faces.

The Government's original proposals to give GPs control of most of the NHS budget and to encourage competition from "any willing provider" have been amended sufficiently to make it likely that the Health and Social Care Bill will be passed by Parliament in the next few months. There remain many other issues to be resolved, of course, including how to commission services from GPs and how to manage the conflicts of interests that GPs will have as being both the purchaser and provider of services. Nevertheless, attention is switching to implementation and how to manage the extraordinarily difficult financial situation.

The problem now, as many critics argue, is that the proposals have been so watered down that they have lost their radical edge and are simply inadequate to deal with the problems. As a result, they believe that the NHS is condemned to a period of attrition where financial considerations will mean that decision making is centralised, services close, standards decline and morale drops. The NHS, it seems, is set for years of managing decline as best it can.

There is an alternative – and we can just begin to see what it looks like. There is already a growing consensus about many aspects of the NHS. There is widespread understanding that the biggest problem the NHS faces is how to care for people with long term and chronic conditions and that it needs to re-design it services accordingly. There is a shared belief that local groups – probably based around GPs – can liberate local creativity and channel community energy and must therefore have a bigger role in planning and decision making. There is also a fair measure of agreement that we need to gather ideas from elsewhere and that the challenge of competition, suitably constrained or regulated, will help bring improvement. In this context the recent expansion of patient choice over service delivery is very welcome.

I believe that this needs to be taken much much further. The logic of all this, as I will argue in the next few pages, is that we need to be clearer about what the NHS is trying to achieve, how it can play its part with other local services in supporting people and communities and how to motivate people and make change happen in a service that employs more than a million people and works with as many more volunteers, family members and paid workers from other organisations.

We can learn something here from the successes and failures of the NHS Plan reforms. Some of this learning is on technical issues. Improvements clearly need to continue in all the four areas of reform I describe in this book – service re-design, system reform, staff re-structuring and access to knowledge, science and technology. However, the most crucial area is in how to motivate people and make change. We got it wrong some of the time with the NHS Plan but we also got it right some of the time.

We can see from the earlier chapters that where it worked there was engagement, local as well as national leadership, clarity of aim and of measurement and accountability and ownership. Where it didn't work was when we relied on purely financial incentives or top-down imposition. Both were resented. Economic incentives can change behaviour but don't motivate and can de-motivate. Like top down instruction they can demean and cheapen.

Neither the Government nor the Opposition seem to me yet to have a clear set of policies or approaches to the reform and improvement of public services – the last Government took at least 4 years before to do so. I believe that study of what happened in the last NHS reforms will be very helpful in developing these ideas; although the new understanding of social networking and social movements that have grown up over the last few years mean that even our most successful methods need to be adapted for the new environment.

This chapter sketches out some ideas about what I think can be done based both on my experience of implementing the NHS reforms, and of subsequently working in other countries.

The challenges

The NHS has come a very long way from the dark days of the 80s and 90s when it was in decline, standards were slipping, A and E was a nightmare and hospital waiting lists stretched into years. The NHS Plan brought the NHS back from the brink. It is stronger than it has been for 30 years or more and enjoys record levels of public satisfaction and cross party political support.[1]

It may have been "saved" but it faces three enormous challenges today.

The first is how to make it sustainable? How can a universal and equitable tax based system be maintained into the future in an era of limited growth and public austerity?

The second is that, despite all the efforts to become more responsive over the last 10 years, the NHS still has a long way to go to become truly patient centred and to listen to patients about what they need.

It has good medical services, good hospitals and primary care and has improved enormously the way that it deals with emergencies and treatments like knee replacements, cataracts, angioplasties and by-pass grafts. These are the more traditional aspects of its work. It is less good at caring for the larger group of people, mostly elderly, who have more complex and long term conditions, and who in recent years have become the biggest users of NHS's resources.

They need continuing help to look after themselves, manage intermittent crises and maintain their health. Despite many excellent examples to the contrary, the NHS is still a service that is geared more towards one-off episodes of treatment.

Moreover, the NHS is still not good enough at listening to patients. The four major Inquiries from Bristol Royal Infirmary to Mid Staffordshire reveal lingering paternalism and protectionism and show how hard it is for the public to make sure that its concerns are heard and acted on. NHS culture, management and regulation still haven't adapted to the idea of a patient led service where what patients think and do is crucially important.

The final challenge is that the NHS still does too little on health promotion and disease prevention. Here again, there are many good things happening, but they are not mainstream.

The opportunity to share in a wider social aim

There is an enormous opportunity here to set the NHS in a new and more sustainable direction. It will require three things: being clear about the aim; building the will and support for its achievement; and creating the means for execution and delivery.

The first of these and the most profound is to start to treat the NHS as what it is – a part of the local infrastructure and services that we all rely on. It should not be seen as a completely separate activity or industry but part of the network of organisations and services locally that help elderly, disabled and sick people to get on with their lives, children to develop, our streets to be safe and our environment and workplaces clean and healthy.

It has its own specific expertise and role but shares in a much wider social aim of helping people to be as independent as possible to live lives they have reason to value in a healthy society and a healthy world.

If we accept this approach we will start to see the problem differently. We will recognise that the NHS budget is part of the wider public and social expenditure locally, that its services need to be integrated with others, staff and facilities linked together, plans merged and assets shared – and that partnership is not an add-on but the central activity. The goal will be integrated local services and not just integrated community health services.

This will reinforce the long standing policy objective of moving from a hospital, professional and treatment based service to a community, people and health based one.

The second action is to build will and a power base for making the necessary changes. This will mean bringing together all the interested parties – the patients' groups, the service providers, the local authorities, the staff interests, the local businesses and the public – to build understanding and the momentum to take on the obstacles in the way and make progress towards achieving the aim. This movement will need to have the power to confront the existing power structures in the NHS which have their interests invested in the status quo. Forward thinking politicians should seize the opportunity to help make this happen.

The third area is to find the new levers and methods that will bring about change. Many are already in existence and there are hundreds of good examples of NHS organisations working in however small a way with other partners on local issues from caring for older people and people with mental illnesses to action on drugs, homelessness and diet. But new mechanisms are also needed to bring the large mainstream NHS budgets into play alongside other local sources of money rather as LIFT has done and social impact bonds have the potential to do.

The absolutely key point here is that is that in searching for innovation, new service models and new providers, the NHS needs to give preference to local organisations, businesses and consortia which in delivering services will also help build local assets and social as well as financial capital.

We need to look for community solutions to communal problems and to open up to any willing and capable **local** provider.

The improvements in the NHS over the last decade and the current high levels of public and political support provide an excellent platform to build on. As importantly, clinicians, managers and policy makers already know most of what needs to be done to redesign services appropriately and are building it into policy and putting it into practice.

What I am proposing is a profound conceptual change but it fits with the developing ideas of the leaders in the NHS and will add energy and impetus to their efforts.

The vision

There is, I believe, a basic vision that most of us would share. We imagine a future where each of us has the opportunity to understand better what will keep us healthy, where we know we can get help when we need it, where care and treatment will be designed for us individually and reflect the full range of our needs, where we and our relatives know what is going on and have choices, where we are confident that our care and treatment will be of reliably high quality and reflect the best evidence and knowledge of the time and where we know that the environment we live in, the food we eat and the society we belong to will all promote our health and not damage it.

It is a future where the NHS works with other local services and with family, neighbours, volunteers and community groups to support us. We don't have to work out individually how to fit into a particular set of services that were designed for everyone but fit very few of us. We don't have to become acutely ill to get help but can be assisted to head-off acute episodes that might otherwise lead to being admitted to hospital. We don't have to explain to the nurse what the doctor said or to struggle to be heard when we tell the clinician that what he or she is proposing has been tried before and didn't work. We don't have to argue with staff about the needs of our elderly relatives or try to convince them that our child isn't over-reacting.

It is a future which is here for some people today where frail and elderly people are able to live in their own homes thanks to intermediate care teams; where disabled people are using individual budgets to design their own services; and where diabetic services for people from South Asian backgrounds reach into the Hindu Temples of the West Midlands to reduce the sugar content of the offerings, promote culturally friendly exercise for women and make it easy for them to accept clinical monitoring and treatment.

It is a future where we aren't, like some of the patients in Mid Staffordshire, "reluctant to insist on receiving basic care or medication for fear of upsetting staff."[2]

Aims – a life we have reason to value

I suspect that most people if asked would describe the aim of the NHS as being about curing illness, helping people be healthy and providing good health services when needed. All of these are of course crucial and what the NHS does daily. I believe, however, that we need to go deeper and wider than this and suggest that the NHS shares in a wider aim to help people to have as much independence as possible so that they can live a life they have reason to value.[*]

This re-definition may at first sight seem both unnecessary and deeply counter intuitive to the professional health worker with many years of education and experience behind them; but in reality it is what most of them do on a daily basis. Many of us by the ages of 50 or 60 have some sort of disability or condition which requires regular attention – whether with statins and other drugs to prevent heart attacks and stroke, insulin to control diabetes or knee, hip and cataract operations to improve the quality of our lives. In all these cases the NHS is clearly helping us to live independently, reduce the burden we might otherwise be on ourselves and others and get the most out of life.

Even with acute conditions – a broken leg, pneumonia or appendicitis – our concern is to recover and "get our lives back". We want "to be able to live at home and independently". Friends with disabilities tell me that they may have to rely on regular healthcare but they want to be treated as individuals in their own right and enabled "to carry on their lives as freely as possible".

Describing the aim in this way emphasises the point that different people value different things and, crucially, that nobody can judge the quality or the value of

---

* I have adapted this from Amartya Sen's discussion of people having "the freedom to live a life they have reason to value" in Development as Freedom, OUP 1999.

someone else's life. Influenced by culture, background, family and personality we make our own choices about health and life even when we are seriously ill or disabled. I have told elsewhere the story of a friend in intensive care who heard doctors saying that she shouldn't be resuscitated because her quality of life was so poor.[3] She was horrified. She would be the judge of her own quality of life.

This point is consistently missed by policy makers. People with a physical disability or illness may be more or less enabled by having or not having family, money, education and community support. They cannot be assessed by the extent of their physical state alone.

This re-definition is also very important because it recognises and gives primacy to the way the NHS has to work with so many other organisations and people – formal organisations like social services and education; informal voluntary and community groups; and relatives, neighbours, friends and carers – as well as the individual themselves in providing care.

There is another aspect, too. Health is connected with everything else in our society. Health and social issues interrelate at every level. The NHS's contribution to society is enormous, helping people back to work, reducing dependency and ill health and having a major impact on the environment, the job market and the economy. Moreover, the NHS is able to work to greatest effect when other services and other parts of society are functioning well. Its particular contribution is to ensure that society is health enhancing and healthy in every sense. Its aims should therefore also embrace the idea of a healthy society.

Finally, we saw in Chapter 2 how the whole world is now interdependent in health terms. We are vulnerable to weaknesses in the health systems of other countries as we saw with SARS and H1N1 which were incubated far away but threatened us along with the rest of the world. Health workers trained in other countries have benefited the NHS as have treatments, drugs and knowledge developed elsewhere. Climate change, nuclear pollution and the health effects of migration affect us all. Health and healthcare are globalising as fast as any other industry or part of society. The NHS has a role to play, too, in sustaining health worldwide.

Taken together these ideas suggest that the NHS should use its expertise in health and healthcare to further the shared aim to:

• enable people to live independently in a way they have reason to value
• support the development of a healthy society
• contribute to the health of an interdependent world.

The NHS has its own specific aims that fit within this wider shared one. I would suggest that these should now be adapted to reflect what IHI calls the Triple Aim – pursuing simultaneously the three aims of improving the experience of care, improving the health of the population and reducing per capita cost of healthcare.[4]

All are important to sustain a national health service available equitably to the whole population.

Building will and a movement for change

The NHS Plan got off to a very good start because it brought together many of the stakeholders around the problems of the time and allowed them to shape some of the solutions – although the Secretary of State wrote the final document. It was launched with widespread support which was maintained over the next two years by bringing stakeholders together in the Modernisation Board. This goodwill and momentum carried the Plan through many difficulties and was helpful when later reforms took the NHS, the Labour Party and much of the public into new territory outside their normal comfort zones.

Something similar is needed here because there will be very difficult issues to deal with. The first and most obvious is that as new services develop they will draw patients away from existing services. Over time there will be less need for large hospital outpatient departments and some services and some whole hospitals will need to close. No one from the local constituency MP onwards relishes the prospect of doing so. Even more profoundly, jobs need to change and in many cases work that was undertaken by highly skilled people can be done by others. Advances in technology will speed this up.

These new services can't just be added to the old but will need to be funded by money withdrawn from the old infrastructure of hospital and outdated clinical and other practices. This is enormously difficult, and as I described in Chapter 5 was not confronted by the politicians during the NHS Plan period when we ended up with more capacity than was needed. We didn't close facilities when we needed to. This contributed to the build up of mistrust and tension between NHS leaders and politicians which eventually replaced the good will evident in 2000.

The second major problem is that the NHS is still a largely hierarchical organisation where some groups are more powerful than others and influence what happens. At the top of the list of the powerful are the doctors and the professional associations, the great hospitals, the research institutes, the universities, the managers and the commercial suppliers of pharmaceuticals and other products.

The way the NHS and other health systems work reflects their interests.[5] These groups mostly earn their living from a system where hospitals and professionals still dominate. There are few incentives for the great teaching hospitals to promote community services, for commerce to encourage cheap low tech solutions and for professional associations to endorse non-professionals taking on wider roles. Even the universities and research institutes earn most of their grant money from developing treatments and not from creating new diagnostic tests or researching health promotion and disease prevention. Most NHS processes and systems from payment systems to clinical training support these interests; although most are already changing to reflect the new reality.

Shifts in power

Governments have for years tried to shift the balance of power through building up GPs and primary care as a counterbalance to the power of Consultants and the hospital sector. A Primary Care Led NHS was announced in the 90s and Alan Milburn and Andrew Lansley have successively announced that 80% of NHS funding would be spent by PCTs and GP consortia respectively.[6, 7] GPs are in many cases now paid more than Consultants and general practice, which was difficult to recruit for at the end of the 90s, is now a speciality of choice for young doctors. There has been some movement as a result, but not yet enough to alter the whole system.

There have been some other shifts in power in the last 60 years as I described in Chapter 2. Over the years the medical power that gained concessions from Bevan has diminished a bit as other professions, most notably nursing, have become stronger and more influential. The Griffiths Report in 1985 created general management as a new NHS power base, designed both to improve the operation of the service but also to begin to hold doctors to account for their activities and expenditure in the NHS.[8]

This managerial approach heralded a new era of managed hospitals, national priorities and, eventually, new contracts, targets and performance management. It brought tensions between doctors and managers as power shifted between them. Politicians backed both sides: extolling doctors as public benefactors whilst demanding managers held them to account. They won friends from neither.

From 2001 the Government began to bring market forces into public services and replace managerial approaches with regulation. It was another power shift and, as I have described in Chapter 5, created tensions for clinicians who wanted to give their patients continuity of care and managers who wanted to plan services effectively. Both feared the fragmentation of services and loss of equity and quality that might result. Both resented the simple over-reliance on economic incentives to deal with the complexities of healthcare.

The time seems to be right to move beyond medical domination, managerialism and markets; keeping the best of each but finding a new model and a new power base in patients, the public and wider society.

Beyond the medical domination, managerialism and the market

One of the lessons from the NHS Plan was the importance of leadership and the effect that coalitions of leaders can have in shaping and implementing improvement. They can also hold the NHS together and hold it to its values during a period of massive uncertainty and change. These shaping and maintaining roles are both needed today.

Such leaders can come from many sources. Nationally there is a new generation of politicians, managers and clinicians who can provide a direction and roles models as a "guiding coalition". How they behave will be critical in holding the NHS together for the next period of its history. The links and relationships between them – and their ability to create relationships with the other national leaders from the patients' groups, professions, universities, local authorities, voluntary organisations, private sector and elsewhere – will be as critical for them in achieving their goals as it was for us. They can learn from our successes as well as our failures.

More locally there are many others including community entrepreneurs, local businesses and many clinicians and professionals from inside health and outside. Many young professional people are passionate about health, society and global issues and will readily identify with the wider aim described here. Most important of all are the patients and the public – who are the only people with the real ability to provide a counterbalance to the power of the professions and the weight of history.

The key point here is that a new "guiding Coalition" must include patients and the public.

Making it happen

There is already a lot happening but it needs to be accelerated.

There are implications in all four of the areas of reform in the NHS Plan. In two of them the implications are straightforward. The processes of system redesign are well advanced. There are now substantial numbers of clinicians and others who have learned techniques of quality improvement. The Quality, Innovation, Productivity and Prevention programme, QIPP, was set up in the Department of Health under the leadership of Jim Easton in 2009 to harness this expertise and help the NHS continue to improve across health services and disease prevention. It needs to reach out even further and connect with local government and others to build locally integrated services across healthcare and beyond.

Similarly, the NHS has a very good foundation in knowledge, science and technology. It has close links with universities and, to a lesser extent, technology and healthcare companies. It also has mechanisms such as the national R and D programme and the National Institute for Health and Clinical Excellence (NICE) to help differentiate the most beneficial innovations and developments from the expensive new versions of therapies and drugs that have marginal additional effect and to disseminate these findings to clinicians.

Over the years there have been many attempts to accelerate the use of appropriate new technology in the NHS with only limited success. These need to be re-doubled but with a changed emphasis to put more focus on the needs of integrated local services and, as I have argued in Chapter 7, on early diagnosis and "early health" rather than late treatment.

IT will undoubtedly have a major beneficial impact in healthcare, although exactly how this will happen has not yet been demonstrated anywhere. There are now some good examples globally although mostly at relatively small scale. The NHS, despite the furore over the IT programme, has as good a national structure at the moment as any other country; but it needs to watch and learn from developments elsewhere and act when the way forward is clear.

Staff restructuring, however, needs major attention. A great deal has been done, with nurses in particular expanding their roles with limited prescribing rights, undertaking more clinical procedures and taking part in some medical rotas. GPs led the biggest change in the variety and nature of roles undertaken by different staff in their practices.

With 60% plus of expenditure in staffing this must be a priority for the NHS and a more planned and radical approach is needed. The staff contracts implemented during the NHS Plan period provide some of the levers that are needed. Financial pressure makes them more likely to be used than they were at a time when resources were freer and difficult decisions easier to avoid. As importantly, the emphasis placed on integrated local services here suggests that there is more scope for changing roles in association with other organisations and developing further the contributions of volunteers, carers and others.

The other major area of change, however, is in system reform. The continuing expansion of Foundation Trusts and the development of payment by results as a more sophisticated model where payments are made for packages of "*best practice*" services are very welcome. So is some distancing of NHS leadership from Ministers. This will allow the Department to focus on public health and wider health issues and give the NHS some freedom from political interference in operational matters.

Two other things are needed. The first is decentralisation of power to a local body. This seems very likely to happen; although whether it will be as GP dominated as the Government originally wanted or has a wider constituency remains to be seen. I think the important feature is that it should not be dominated either by the doctors and other professions or any other interest group. Whatever its constituents it needs to have the same remit as PCTs for commissioning services, promoting public health and developing primary and community care.

The second thing, which isn't yet happening, is the development of ways to integrate more fully local services, local budgets and local investment – with the NHS as a full participant – and the introduction of a requirement that preference should be given to locally based organisations in funding developments and commissioning services.

Let me illustrate what I mean with one example of current activity from many that I could have chosen.

Integrated local services and "inside out" thinking

The keys to successful local partnerships and community enterprise as Lord Andrew Mawson, the social entrepreneur, has pointed out are people and relationships not committees and processes.

Andrew's own work started more than 25 years ago in Bromley by Bow in East London and provides a very good example of what can be done. Starting with no more than a church hall and a few parishioners he built up a network of local activities – from dance classes to a pre-school playgroup, to providing premises for a health centre and GP practice to arts activities to employment schemes.[9] Over time – and only after much difficulty – the authorities began to engage him in their re-development plans, revitalising local schools and other facilities and now there is a thriving set of small social and business enterprises in the community with £1 billion of investment under local management.

He argues that this wasn't achieved by top down or bottom up activity but by "inside out" thinking – by which he meant that it depended on identifying the assets in the community and building on them.

He gave examples of these assets from his own experience: like the pharmacist who would be willing to mentor school children interested in a career in pharmacy, the school and his own church which were unused most of the time, the potential to engage entrepreneurs and professional people living locally in local activities, the opportunity to give a local dance teacher the start she needed to set up a business, the nursery which was self funding because wealthier residents as well as the less well off sent their children there. These assets could all be put to use. Now there is a thriving community of people engaged with each other and building a healthier society, supported by new facilities created jointly by different organisations.

The inside out concept is a very important switch in emphasis from the thinking of the planners and the professionals we all recognise – where people can't do something because there isn't another x or enough y or because it doesn't match some theoretical model of good practice drawn up by experts. Traditional thinking focuses on what you don't have; inside out thinking concentrates on what you do.

Inside out thinking fits very well with the processes of quality improvement with their focus on improving the system – making the bits work better together – and making improvements without any extra cost. As we shall see in the next chapter, the most enterprising and successful leaders and innovators in low and middle income countries use the assets to hand to deliver what they need to deliver.

The inside out thinking resonated strongly with the leaders from many sectors of the Sheffield community – University, Police, City Council, Fire and Rescue

Service, business and health – who were brought together recently by Chris Liddle of HLM Architects. In discussion they described similar but smaller examples around their City. Their task as they saw it was to use the £1.8 billion of public money spent annually to best effect; each sharing assets and opportunities with each other.

We were in the City Hall and Andrew went on to remind us that cities like Sheffield were built by the entrepreneurs of the industrial revolution. As he summoned up the shades of the pioneers of a very different age he suggested that today's social and business entrepreneurs could provide a lot of the energy and creativity we now need.

There is an interesting reflection here on the role of private enterprise. In the Mawson model small businesses and entrepreneurs work alongside other local people and organisations to create value locally. It is not the big organisations and healthcare chains from the UK and America coming in to support GPs or run services. Crucially, those organisations' headquarters are elsewhere and they have no stake locally. It is about local people and businesses working with local authorities and contributing to local regeneration and development. Such groupings have re-built so many of our town and city centres and even in health we have the example of Local Improvement Finance Trusts (LIFT) partnerships to show how this can be done.

LIFT partnerships (see Chapter 7) are designed as partnerships between NHS organisations and businesses which, based on the strategic plan for the area, invest in new community and primary care premises. A recent review noted that:

> "LIFT is a partnership which should be based on confidence and trust. There should be a movement away from the client and contractor mode which would normally be in existence in both the public and private sector for capital procurements."[10]

It is a powerful statement of working through relationships and people and, interestingly, goes on to say that that the quality of relationships has significantly determined which LIFT partnerships were successful and which weren't.

This discussion brings into focus the differences between economic and business thinking. A large part of the NHS Plan reforms were based on economic thinking about incentives. I described in Chapter 6 how economic incentives influence clinicians and others in the health service but only up to a point – the one dimensional notion of rational economic man doesn't apply in health anymore than it applies elsewhere. People have other motivations. There are limits to markets. The business thinking shared by private and social entrepreneurs is different and is about what you can do with the assets to hand. It is about people actively doing something not just responding to incentives.

LIFT is a very interesting example because it shows how new arrangements can be developed that support local endeavour across organisational boundaries. It really only deals with premises and some equipment but suggests the possibility that similar models could be developed to deal with wider issues including service provision, infrastructure development, the introduction of new technologies and staff training.

The development of social impact bonds by the previous and the current Government is just such a very promising model – whereby money is raised through philanthropy or venture capitalists to fund a social programme with the investors only getting a return if there is a social impact. The report *"Early Intervention: Smart Investment, Massive Savings"* published in July 2011 promises to take this further.

These possibilities for shared ventures between the NHS and local businesses and other organisations and shared working with local enterprises and authorities offer enormous scope for innovation. The Department has spent a great deal of time and effort in working through how GPs – with their investments in their practices as small businesses – can take the leading role locally. It can use some of the same thinking to develop new arrangements to let others play a wider role. It needs to do so in such a way as to avoid the constraints of European competition and procurement law and permit preference to be given to locally based enterprises with a stake in the community.

Sustainability

The NHS is facing a profound squeeze. It has had an average 5.5% annual real growth for 10 years. Even in the previous 20 years – when it was in decline – real growth averaged 3.1%. The next four years will see virtually no growth.

It will no doubt return to growth in the longer term. The long term trend has been for societies to increase health spending by about 1.1% for every 1% of growth in GDP. The UK is well placed financially in health compared to most other similar countries. It still spends below the European average on health and spends 25% less than either France or Germany – spending less from the public purse as well as from private sources. In a recent authoritative comparison with similar nations it came top on effective care, efficiency and cost related barriers to care; second on access, safe care and equity and second in overall performance.[11]

In the meantime, however, there is a widespread feeling that the NHS and other universal public systems can only survive by restricting the services they cover and by patients paying more.[12, 13] These responses will tend to reduce the NHS to the status of an insurer. It has until now been a social contract between citizen and state with an expectation that NHS staff and organisations will always try to do their best for each patient and where decision making is open to scrutiny. The NHS Constitution with all Party support reinforces this wider role.[14] It is not a commercial contract with all the exclusions and limitations that that implies.

I believe that we need to act decisively now to avoid this counsel of despair. There is, however, nothing easy about this and no sure formula for success; but some combination of the following would seem to be the best approach.

Firstly, the scale of the problem needs to be understood and confronted. The processes I have described of redefining aim, building will and developing new approaches need to be followed through.

These have many parts as we have seen. They require rigorously ensuring that as new more integrated local services are developed funding is extracted from the old infrastructure and old practices. At the same time the approaches I advocate for bringing budgets together, "inside out" thinking and finding new sources of investment offer greater scope for making existing finances go further, as does continuing scrutiny of evidence for effectiveness and cost effectiveness. The Triple Aim approach will aid coordination and planning and ensure a focus on the most important issues.

Secondly, the existing work being led by QIPP and the financial demands made by Sir David Nicholson need to be firmly orientated towards making the desirable service and infrastructure changes – taking into account the wider picture beyond the NHS – with support given to some of the more difficult changes where the case for making them is clear. It is encouraging to see David and other leaders, including the General Secretary of the Royal College of Nursing, arguing that some services will have to be centralised and some hospitals closed. Politicians need to help support them. Sadly, there is already evidence that some people are taking the easier option of "rationing" services.

Thirdly, a new analysis of the type undertaken by Derek Wanless in 2002 needs to be made of future demand and costs and setting out, as he did, what the different scenarios will look like.[15] However, unlike what happened with the Wanless Review, I would suggest that its findings are opened up for wider discussion and debate before decisions are made by the government of the day. This can provide the basis around which patients, professionals and the public can come together to work for change.

Fourthly, the intellectual arguments need to be well made and the myths dispelled. It is worth remembering that there are many interested parties who would like the NHS to restrict its services and increase payments for patients. Private insurers and health providers and everyone involved in private medicine and supplying medical products have an interest in seeing their markets expand and expenditure grow.

There are four common and dangerous myths. One is that demand for healthcare is infinite. It isn't, but supply is. The professions and commercial interest can always think of extra services and interventions. Many patients, however, don't seek healthcare when they need it and the NHS often has to seek them out. Many of us avoid doctors or hospitals! A second is that NHS healthcare is free. It isn't.

There are often enormous costs in the time and effort of patients and their relatives and carers in seeking help.

Thirdly, healthcare is sometimes treated only as a cost, whereas economic analysis shows clearly that good health benefits the economy with an American estimate suggesting that half of GDP growth from 1970 to 2000 was due to improved health.[16] Conversely, other sources suggest that the AIDS epidemic has reduced South African growth by 1% per annum. Fourthly, there seems to be an implicit assumption that innovation only comes from the private for profit sector – which when written down this baldly needs no answer because it is so obviously wrong.

Somewhere and somehow through this combination of activities – and if the political will is there – the NHS can not only remain saved but be put on a more sustainable footing for the future. The country does have choices about how much it spends on healthcare and about whether it wants to live up to the old ambition that everyone should have access to good healthcare "regardless of their ability to pay".

It is an aspiration worthy of any Government or society.

References

1. Social attitudes survey.
2. Mid Staffordshire NHS Foundation Trust Inquiry Final report; February 2010, para 14.
3. Nigel Crisp (2010) *Turning the World Upside Down*, RSM Press, Jan.
4. Berwick DM, Nolan TW, Whittington J (2008) The Triple Aim: Care, Health, And Cost. *Health Affairs* **27**(3): 759–69.
5. Ivan Illich (1976) *The limits to Medicine. Medical nemesis: the appropriation of health*, Marion Boyars.
6. Alan Milburn, Shifting the balance of power, speech April 2001.
7. Health and Social Care Bill, 2010-2011.
8. Sir Roy Griffiths: Griffiths Report – NHS Management Inquiry; Department of Health; 1983.
9. Andrew Mawson (2008) *The Social Entrepreneur*, Atlantic Books.
10. Department of Health (2008) *Review of LIFT (Local Investment Finance Trusts) carried out by Caroline Rassell*, Nov.
11. The Commonwealth Health Fund (2010) *Mirror, mirror on the wall: how the performance of the US health system compares internationally*, update.
12. Jeremy Laurance (2010) From wheelchairs to new breasts – what should the NHS pay for? *Independent* 8 March.
13. Economist Intelligence Unit: *The future of healthcare in Europe*; 2011.
14. Department of Health (2010) *The NHS Constitution: securing the NHS today for generations to come*, 8 March.
15. Derek Wanless (2002) *Our future health: taking a long term view*, HM Treasury, April.
16. Murphy KM, Topel RH (2006) The value of health and longevity. *Journal of Political Economy* **114**(5): 871–904.

Chapter 13

Reforming and strengthening health systems around the world

Last year I flew to Brazil to join the South Africa Health Minister, Dr Aaron Motsoaledi, who had gone there with a team of senior colleagues to learn about the health system.

It was very instructive. Brazil and South Africa have similar levels of GDP, both have enormous inequalities between rich and poor in their populations and both are now fast developing BRICS countries. Brazil made health a national priority more than 10 years ago and has persevered with improvement ever since. It has a particularly impressive record of developing primary care services for its far flung rural population. South Africa is setting out on a similar journey and seeking to learn from others wherever it can.

It was a very good demonstration that all countries can learn from the experiences of each other – and a salutary reminder that the rich and highly developed countries don't have all the answers.

Everyone has something to teach and everyone has something to learn

This chapter sets out what I think other countries may be able to learn from our experience with the NHS Plan reforms. I put these ideas forward very modestly, recognising both that nothing can be simply transferred from one country to another – context and environment are crucial to success – and that new ideas are being developed in many low and middle income countries that are very relevant to the UK.[1] Knowledge transfer is two way.

Most high income countries have very developed health systems, which like the UK, are very heavily invested in hospitals, highly trained professionals and a treatment approach to health. Most are struggling with similar issues about how to manage financial pressures whilst continuing to improve, how to cope with growing demand from an ageing population and how to move towards a more community and prevention based health service.

Many of these countries have taken an economic focus to reform, concentrating on changing financial flows, insurance and payment systems. I would argue, however, that as in the UK they need to clarify what their health systems are really trying to achieve and to redefine their ultimate aim in a similar way as being about their citizens and society. Many may also be well served by adopting a *Triple Aim* type approach of the sort I described in the last chapter. It will change the way they conceive of their health system and, potentially, bring new assets into play.

Most of these countries, like the UK, have introduced changes in all the four areas of reform I have described in this book but have done least in the area of staff re-structuring. It is the most difficult area and the one where there will be most opposition to change.

Low and middle income countries

Whilst these richer countries may find some aspects of our approach – and our successes and failures – useful as they plan the next stages of their reform and try to make their systems sustainable, I will concentrate in this chapter on low and middle income countries. They face far worse health problems and rather different issues. They have weak systems which need to be built up rather than strong ones which need to be reformed and are mostly focussing their efforts on achieving the Millennium Development Goals (MDGs) of reducing maternal and child mortality and tackling the killers of HIV/AIDS, TB and malaria.[2]

In the UK it is sometimes difficult to comprehend the health problems in other countries. I described earlier how Sub Saharan Africa has 10% of the world's population and 25% of the burden of disease but only 1.5% of the world's health workers to deal with it. To put this in perspective it is like trying to deal with all the patients who use one of our large UK hospitals with less than 2% of the staff. St Thomas's might have eight doctors, Addenbrookes 12, the whole of Newcastle 30 and Manchester 75. In China an admission to a University Hospital costs 80% of the average annual wage.[3] In the UK an NHS hip operation costs about 20% of the average annual wage. The patient would have to pay personally in China. The operation would be free in the UK.

Looking forward, low and middle income countries with weak and underdeveloped systems have the opportunity as they grow to leap frog over the UK and other richer countries and create new types of more community based systems. They don't need to repeat our development path and can learn from our mistakes. In the short term, however, they are struggling with enormous problems.

China, India and other countries are actively involved in developing their health systems. Other countries like Pakistan are working to develop what they have – much of it inherited from British colonialism – whilst others like Ethiopia are essentially building from the ground up.[4] "*Health systems strengthening*" has become a key theme in international development. The experience of the NHS Plan with its emphasis on systems and targets for improvement may have something to offer.

It is likely to be particularly relevant in those countries where, like the UK, Government is the main actor in health systems as planner, funder and, often, provider. Most Commonwealth countries have such systems which were modelled on the 1948 NHS.

The experience of the NHS Plan reforms

There were a number of essential starting points for the reforms.

The first was that the NHS was born after the Second World War as part of the re-building of the country. It was a component of the Welfare State which embraced education, employment and social security as well as health. Many low and middle income countries have development plans for their whole countries covering the economy, poverty reduction and social development. They too are very often in the process of rebuilding their countries and societies after war or other catastrophic events. Health fits within these wider aspirations.

This background helps shape the aim of the health service. As I have argued in earlier chapters this aim needs to be about using health and healthcare expertise to help people to be independent to live a life they have reason to value as part of a healthy society and a healthy world. It can be very tempting to think that building up a health system simply means creating more hospitals and training more professionals. This can be very beguiling. Politicians, the media and the public may well see these as symbols of progress – and, indeed, more and better hospitals and professionals will surely be needed. Many leaders, however, understand fully that they need to build up the whole infrastructure and engage all sectors of the economy and population in their efforts.

The NHS Plan was launched with great energy and widespread support. It captured the aspirations of many people and created a momentum that helped carry it through later difficulties. It had cross Government support – including the Finance Ministry – and the personal support of the leader of the Government. These are vital features for successful health developments, as the Brazilian and other experiences also demonstrate.[5]

It set out clear and measurable objectives. There was nothing vague about its targets, although there were, initially at least, too many of them. We were also able to create a very effective implementation process which delivered very significant and substantial results.

Results took time, however, and there was an anxious period of more than a year before we could see progress – and then it was very slight at first. This is likely to be a common pattern and efforts need to be made to have some "quick wins" and other morale boosting initiatives to maintain momentum and show that there is sufficient will and determination to see this through. I was told "we didn't think you were serious about reducing waiting until the second year". We showed we were – year on year for 10 years.

There were also temptations to relax once improvements started to come. I was asked "*my waiting list is down to 6 months, isn't that good enough?*" No, it wasn't. Transformational change takes time, perseverance and attention to detail. Good plans and designs for reform are important but can't replace the day to day grind of delivery.

We also started with an excellent quality framework. We had a system for assessing organisations and quality assuring performance: through the Commission for Healthcare Improvement, later replaced by the Commission for Health and Care Quality Commission and supported by other organisations to deal with doctor's performance and other aspects of quality. We had in the National Institute for Health and Clinical Excellence (NICE) a system for assessing technologies which later developed systematic approaches for making clinical evidence available across the NHS. We had regulators for the professions, designed to protect patients; although later events showed that we needed to reform these.

I have observed in a number of countries that Governments have concentrated on only some aspects of this framework, with many dealing only with quality assurance and inspection controls. These are obviously important but, I would suggest, insufficient.

Whilst these features gave us an excellent framework within which to make improvement they did not in themselves guarantee improvement. We also needed good quality improvement methods and management processes to make anything actually happen.

Quality improvement and management – delivery

I described in Chapter 4 how we developed a two handed approach to delivery. On the one hand we made sure there were clear accountability arrangements in place and that we held people to account both personally and in public by creating league tables, giving star ratings and insisting that quality, financial and other results were published. It was a tough regime.

On the other hand we developed quality improvement approaches and spread good practice, initially through the Modernisation Agency. Over time we have built up a large number of clinicians and others who understand and can apply these methodologies and the legacy lives on in England through QIPP, the NHS Institute and other more local programmes.

An important part of the learning here has been to think of the health system as genuinely a system where changes in one part can affect another. Making improvement therefore isn't about just putting in more inputs – such as staff or facilities – but about making the system work better. More inputs are of course needed in many cases but how they are used is essential. More resources wrongly deployed can turn a cheap poorly performing service into an expensive poorly performing one. Using system methods to improve health systems is vital.

The World Health Organisation (WHO) set out a model for systems strengthening which looked like it was mainly concerned with the building blocks of a system and not with how the parts worked together. A later research paper "*Systems thinking for health systems strengthening*", however, corrected the balance.[6]

There is now a great deal of activity around health systems research with new institutes, conferences and publications springing up around the world. It looks at last as if quality improvement as used for years by a few organisations like IHI in the US and elsewhere, URC around the world and the MA in England may move towards the centre of the stage in development.

There were of course dangers and problems in what we did in England as I have described in earlier chapters. The very strong political and central leadership sometimes meant that we didn't hear what people were saying. We missed the importance of MRSA in 2000 and had to come back to it 2003, catching up for lost time. We sometimes got the balance wrong between the management and the improvement approach and we certainly underestimated problems with some major projects. All these issues need to be identified as risks, watched for and managed.

Our processes were very much part of the local context. Whilst I suspect this management/improvement balance has universal relevance, its application must be local.

In turning to the four areas of reform I will try to address in particular the problems I have been alerted to in meetings in Africa, China and India – drawing out any relevant learning from our experience. My observation is that these four areas of reform are themselves as relevant in these countries as they are in the UK and that progress is needed in all of them.

Service redesign

I have already touched on service redesign in this chapter and described it more extensively earlier. It was developed as an approach in healthcare by the Massachusetts based IHI, borrowing from other industries, and initially applied in high income countries and hospital based systems. In recent years IHI and URC have demonstrated that it can be effective in resource-poor countries and community settings. The principles of improvement are universal.

Figure 13.1 shows the improvements made in the number of mothers receiving appropriate prenatal care in Ecuador by using these methods.[7] It is one of many such compelling examples from around the world.

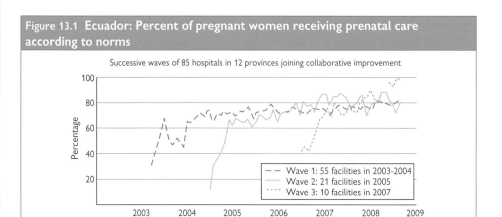

Figure 13.1 **Ecuador: Percent of pregnant women receiving prenatal care according to norms**

System reform

As in the UK, service redesign is important but not sufficient to transform healthcare. There also need to be changes in the way the whole system works in order to accelerate and embed improvement.

I believe, as I have said, that this needs to start with defining the aim of the system – being clear about what it is trying to do. It is interesting to note that in Bangladesh the very large voluntary organisation BRAC provides healthcare alongside education, micro finance loans and much else for the poor of the country. It doesn't see health as a separate industry, divorced from everything else. It also involves and engages family, women and the community in planning and delivering services for themselves and their neighbours.

I have argued elsewhere that some low and middle income countries are developing new sorts of health systems, more integrated into their local communities, making use of the assets at hand – using "inside out" thinking as Andrew Mawson described it in the last chapter – blending public health and treatment and training people for the tasks in hand not just for the professions.[8] We have a great deal to learn.

Underneath what I have described as the shared aim, I think that many countries may want to adapt the concept of the Triple Aim, again described in the last chapter, as an operational aim for its health system.[9] This would mean simultaneously pursuing the three aims of improving the experience of care, improving the health of populations and reducing per capita costs of healthcare. In low and middle income countries where there is an obvious need for massive investment the third aim might more appropriately be to manage per capita costs of healthcare to what is affordable at the time.

Each of these aims is individually important; pursued simultaneously they offer the hope of a sustainable health system.

I have already commented on the importance of a quality framework as part of the system, shaping its development and guiding its performance. This needs to link with building strong accountability, creating a management framework and decentralising authority to local level – whatever form that might take in the particular country.

In recent discussions in China on behalf of the China Medical Board I was told how weak such management systems were locally and how difficult devolution was. I told them that we started out on this journey in 1985 with the introduction of General Managers, followed this up by creating NHS trusts with their own boards in 1991, gave NHS Foundation Trusts greater legal autonomy in 2002 and still have little more than half the country covered by them. This is a very long journey.

The Chinese and many others see the development of primary care as a fundamental part of their reform strategy to provide good local care, to reduce the burden on hospitals and provide a counter balance to the power of the specialists and acute hospitals. Their approach cannot be the same as ours, although they may wish to understand and draw ideas from our experience. This too has been a very long march with General Practice becoming a speciality alongside others only in 1952 – the Royal College of Physicians dates back 500 years – and there have been many subsequent developments in training and role to establish the high quality service and increasing powerful primary care sector we have today.

Many systems like the English NHS are opening up to the private sector and some like Kenya for example have for years had many of their services provided by local and international foundations, NGOs and charities. The English experience may be helpful as an example of how we maintained NHS values, quality standards and identity whilst offering people the opportunity to be NHS patients in private facilities. We saw evidence that increased internal and external competition improved services. We also developed a process through the Care Quality Commission to approve and inspect public and private service providers on essentially the same basis.

The NHS introduced a payment by results approach for paying service providers for their activity. Again we have been on a development path, starting with some relatively crude categorisation of activity and pricing 8 years ago but now having developed "best practice" categories to ensure that this pricing mechanism helps to drive the improvements that are wanted.

The NHS has a single payer and is tax funded and therefore has no relevant experience in insurance systems. However, our experience of the Private Finance Initiative which we used to provide more than £15 billion of investment in both secondary and primary care may be useful.

What is very evident in all these areas of system reform is that other countries may very well be able to speed up their own processes of development by studying ours. In many cases they may be able to "leap frog" our developments.

Staff restructuring

The UK and other countries can learn more about staff restructuring from low and middle income countries than the other way round. In many countries health leaders have instituted training programmes for mid-level workers who perform technical tasks and undertake surgery and other procedures more usually done by doctors or other professionals. Under the right conditions they can be as successful as doctors at certain procedures, cost much less and – very importantly in countries affected by migration – remain locally rather than joining many professional people in emigrating.[10]

In many countries these sorts of arrangements are seen as temporary expedients and only tolerated until more money and staff enable the education and employment of professionals. I believe that this can be a mistake. There is a need, of course, for very highly trained health workers and scientists at the top of the staffing pyramid in any country. In some cases, semi-skilled and part trained people are trying to work completely outside their competences and do need to be replaced or trained appropriately when resources are available.

However, this does not mean that countries should copy our top heavy staffing structures. Indeed, where it is clear that mid-level workers are performing as well as much more expensive and expensively trained professionals there is every incentive for countries to keep them and for others to copy the approach. Good healthcare can be provided by lower qualified people under the right conditions.

England does have some relevant experience of widening the role of nurses in particular – with nurse prescribing, nurse endoscopists and nurse Consultants – and introducing new grades of staff such as imaging and vascular technicians. Other countries will, like the UK, have to deal with very reasonable professional concerns about quality and with, sometimes unreasonable, trade unionism in these areas.

In some countries there is very little regulation and development is needed. In others such as South Africa health worker regulation appears to be too restrictive and rigid. In India I observed that the Medical Association is even more territorial and conservative than the BMA and keen to control all developments.

We have had to fight some of the battles which these countries must endure – and we will have more to come.

Knowledge, technology and science

Here again, there is some scope for richer countries to learn from some of the experience of low and middle income countries where the absence of pre-existing infrastructure can lead to developments skipping a generation so that, for example, telemedicine is developing faster and going further in low and middle countries than in richer ones.

Looking at the English experience I think there are two main areas of interest for other countries. The first is NICE with its developed techniques for assessing new technologies and providing evidence to the service. It has had so much interest from other countries that it is now setting up an international arm to cope. The second is in the way that the Department has brought together over the last few years leaders from the NHS, the civil service, universities, research institutes and commerce around R and D to gain better mutual understanding and look for synergies and alignment. It is providing England with a good foundation for moving ahead scientifically.

Expenditure and sustainability

Ariel Pablos-Mendez and colleagues have shown that there is an "economic transition" when countries reach a point in their growth at which they start to aspire to universal health coverage for their population and where they can begin to afford it.[11] They also note that healthcare costs are on a long term upward trajectory that correlates very closely with growing GDP and cite Baumol's description of health and education suffering from a "cost disease" because as very labour-intensive industries they will tend to experience higher inflation than many others.[12]

Taken together these points all raise questions for countries as to how they will develop their health systems and whether they will broadly follow an American type private insurance model or a European "social solidarity". Some like the Chinese have tried one – the American – but more recently converted to the European as costs got out of hand and their population demanded improvement.

Most countries can only progress step by step: as resources become available they are able to expand their healthcare offering to more conditions and more of the population. There may well be some lessons here from England where a tax based universal system is based firmly on primary care where GPs act as gatekeepers to the secondary sector; where payment by results is just maturing into a system which can help channel funding to priority activities; where the private sector provides some competition for public sector providers and the Private Finance Initiative has accelerated investment in new infrastructure.

Ultimately, however, choices about the way healthcare is funded and provided are very dependent on cultural and social norms and perspective. We can expect that new ideas and new business models will develop in low and middle income countries – as they already have with eye care where Aravind in India cross subsidises care for the poor from the fees paid by the better off.

The future needs to be about sharing our experiences and our insights. Everyone has something to teach and everyone has something to learn.

References

1. Nigel Crisp (2010) *Turning the World Upside Down – the search for global health in the 21st century*; RSM Press, Jan.

2. See website on Millennium Development Goals for full list.

3. Analysis reported to me by Professor Gordon G Liu of Peking University, April 2011.

4. Nishtar S (2010) *Choked Pipes: Reforming Pakistan's Mixed Health System*. Oxford University Press.

5. Crisp N, Gawanas B, Sharp I (2008) *Scaling up, Saving lives*. Global Health Workforce Alliance.

6. World Health Organisation (2009) *Systems thinking for health systems strengthening*. WHO, Geneva.

7. Franco LM, Marquez L, Ethier K, Balsara Z, Isenhower W (2009) *Results of Collaborative Improvement: Effects on Health Outcomes and Compliance with Evidence-based Standards in 27 Applications in 12 Countries*, USAID Dec, p 4.

8. Nigel Crisp (2010) *Turning the World Upside Down – the search for global health in the 21st century*, RSM Press, Jan.

9. Berwick DM, Nolan TW, Whittington J (2008) The Triple Aim: Care, Health, And Cost. *Health Affairs* **27**(3): 759–69.

10. Kruk ME, Pereira C, Vaz F, Bergström S, Galea S (2007). Economic evaluation of surgically trained assistant medical officers in performing major obstetric surgery in Mozambique. *Br J Obstet Gynaecol* **114**: 1253–60.

11. Pablos-Mendez A, Brown H, de Ferranti D. *"Cost disease" and the economic transition of Global Health*; to be published.

12. WJ Baumol (1993) Social wants and dismal science: the curious case of the climbing costs of health and teaching. *Proc AM Philos Soc* **137**: 612–37.

Chapter 14

The global challenge

In 1999 almost every country in the world signed up to the Millennium Development Goals and committed themselves to delivering improvement globally in the reduction of deaths of young children, pregnant women and children and to reducing infections from HIV/AIDS, malaria, TB and other communicable diseases by 2015.[1] It was a bold and ambitious statement of everyone's right to health and of global interdependence.

Enormous improvements have been made but the goals aren't going to be met in every country in the world and the targeted reductions in maternal mortality won't be achieved for the globe as a whole. The barriers have been social as much as about clinical practice and resources. Women and poor people have little access to healthcare and poor women have the least of all. It is not just about economics but about culture, exclusion and power.

The Commission on the Social Determinants of Health has anatomised the situation and demonstrated the relationships between position in society and ill health.[2] Power sets the agenda on health globally as on everything else and behind the statistics of mortality and morbidity lie other statistics about which parts of the world share in trade, in foreign direct investment and in agreements that protect their interests. The global development organisations, almost always peopled by decent and idealistic people, have all too often reinforced the hegemony with inappropriate policies and casual assumptions about who knows best.

The world is beginning to change. In 2011 South Africa joined the BRICS in a grouping that covers more than 40% of the world's population and more than 20% of its economy. It and the G20, starting to replace G7 and G8, are fast becoming more powerful and will soon be re-writing some of the global rules.

In health the development partners, whether they are the big national agencies like USAID or the UK's DFID or the global initiatives like GAVI and the Global Fund, have adopted a new and more respectful approach in recent years and tried to support "country led development". Nevertheless they still dominate much of the global dialogue about development and are very influential in shaping the way health systems are developing globally. They still mostly carry with them assumptions learned in the rich countries of the world about what is needed in the low and middle income countries. Given the problems in those richer countries, this must surely stop.

Looking forward and taking account of some of the lessons from the NHS Plan reforms I believe that the World Health Organisation (WHO) and other global leaders need to shift their stance and behaviour in two key respects. The first is to build ever stronger their links with all the other parts of the UN family that are concerned with society and improvement and development. Health can no longer be an isolated industry, speaking its own language and dealing only with its own concerns.

The second is to treat the whole world as one place where discussions about health affect us all without separating out the advantaged from the disadvantaged. We are all aware that Sub Saharan Africa has so many more problems than most others, but we can all learn about health systems and community services from each other. As Chief Executive of the NHS I barely noticed the WHO, rather assuming that with the exception of SARS and other communicable diseases it was only concerned with low and middle income countries. It was for the enthusiasts and the specialists.

I believe that there are now, however, some specific things it and others can do to promote better health for us all. Three stand out. The first is to promote the role of quality improvement as the main method of implementing change alongside management in any health system. The evidence is now there for this approach. The second is to begin to collect the evidence of how integrated local services which engage patients and the public as well as professionals – as opposed to integrated community health services – can play an important role in health.

Underpinning both of these is the human resources agenda driven by the Global Health Workforce Alliance and WHO's human resources department. Far too little research is done on human resources, which is surprising given that staff costs are typically about 60% of healthcare costs. Staff restructuring is under-developed in richer countries and it can't any more be treated simply as being about "task shifting" in low and middle income ones.

This also involves developing and implementing new models of professional education as exemplified by the recent Independent Global Commission report on the education of health professionals (of which I was a member) that advocates a system of education based on health systems and inter- and trans-professional learning which would require far greater understanding of society, a focus on teamwork and on transformative learning.[3]

Leadership and management of health systems

This book gives my personal account of running a massive national system during a period of reform. It shows what we set out to do and describes some of the successes and failures.

It was not straightforward and clear cut. Little actions ripple out, producing as many unintended consequences as intended ones. Paradoxes abound. It is as important to be consistent and send clear messages as it is to be adaptable to changed circumstances and new evidence. The two aren't always compatible. The priorities of the health system may sometimes clash with those of other systems and may not fit with the imperatives of politics and public perceptions. The media and the multiplicity of players complicate and enrich the task.

There is as yet little research on managing health systems and relatively little taught about it in our universities and institutions. It is a matter of growing importance as we begin to understand that systems thinking and leadership holds the key to much of the improvement we can make in health and healthcare.

I hope that this account will offer insight and encourage others to contribute their thoughts and experiences so that we can all learn from them.

References

1. MDGs.
2. World Health Organisation (2008) *Closing the gap in a generation: Health equity through action on the social determinants of health*; Commission on Social Determinants of Health.
3. Frenk J, Chen L, Bhutta ZA, *et al* (2010) Health professionals for a new century: transforming education to strengthen health systems in an interdependent world. *The Lancet* **376**(9756): 1923–58.

Appendix 1

Glossary and abbreviations

A and E/Accident and Emergency Department – hospital emergency department

BMA/British Medical Association – medical trade union

CHI/Commission for Health Improvement and CHAI/Commission for Healthcare Audit and Inspection (The Healthcare Commission) – successively the healthcare quality inspector which issued star ratings and later annual report cards, see CQC

Clinician – doctor, nurse or other person who provides direct treatment for patients

Consultant – most senior hospital doctor under whose care a patient is admitted to hospital

CQC/Care Quality Commission – replaced CHAI and the Social Services Inspectorate in 2008 to cover both health and social care and with wider powers of regulation across the public and private sectors

FCE/Finished Consultant Episode – a period of admission to hospital under the care of a Consultant, the normal unit used for payment to hospitals

Foundation Trust – see NHS Foundation Trust

GMC/General Medical Council – medical regulator that approves the registration of doctors allowed to practice in the UK

GP/General Practitioner – doctor who works in primary care, normally working in a practice shared with other doctors and with a registered list of patients under their care

Junior doctor/doctor in training – qualified doctor who is undergoing initial post registration training or training for a speciality, including general practice

Health Authority – body responsible for the health of a population: Regional HA, District HA, Area HA, Strategic HA at different times and with different roles

IHI/Institute for Healthcare Improvement – global leader in quality improvement based in Cambridge, Massachusetts

LIFT/Local Investment Finance Trust – local joint venture between Government and investors to fund development of primary and community facilities

MA/Modernisation Agency and National Institute for Innovation and Improvement/the NHS Institute – agencies established successively to identify and spread best practice using quality improvement methods

Monitor – independent regulator of NHS Foundation Trusts

NHS/National Health Service – established under the NHS Act 1946 to provide comprehensive healthcare for the people of the UK regardless of the ability to pay

NHS Foundation Trust – NHS service provider established from 2003 independent of NHS accountability and regulated by Monitor

NHS Trust – NHS service provider established from 1991 with own Board but remaining accountable to NHS Chief Executive and Government

NICE/National Institute for Clinical and Health Excellence – independent body set up to assess new therapies in the NHS and now providing wide range of clinical guidelines and making evidence available to NHS

PBR/payment by results – method of paying service provider for services

PCT/Primary Care Trust – established in three waves from 2000 to commission services, promote public health and develop primary care. Replaced most local layer of Health Authorities from 2002

Permanent Secretary – the most senior official in a government department, part of the permanent civil service

PFI/Private Finance Initiative – method of providing private finance for investment in NHS facilities

Public Health – concerned with the health of a population with main focus on prevention of disease and promotion of health rather than treatment

Royal College – Statutory Body that promotes standards, quality and training within the particular speciality concerned

Royal College of Nursing – part concerned as other Royal Colleges with standards and quality but also has Trade Union function

Secretary of State – Senior Minister responsible for a Department, member of Cabinet

Trust – see NHS Trust and NHS Foundation Trust

Waiting list – patients waiting either for attendance at an outpatient consultation or, having been seen by a doctor, for admission to hospital

Appendix 2

Structure of the NHS

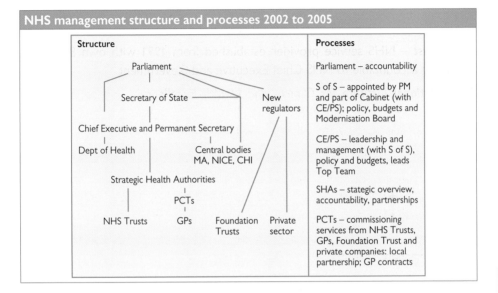

NHS management structure and processes 2002 to 2005

Structure	Processes
Parliament	Parliament – accountability
Secretary of State — New regulators	S of S – appointed by PM and part of Cabinet (with CE/PS); policy, budgets and Modernisation Board
Chief Executive and Permanent Secretary	
Dept of Health — Central bodies MA, NICE, CHI	CE/PS – leadership and management (with S of S), policy and budgets, leads Top Team
Strategic Health Authorities	
PCTs	SHAs – stategic overview, accountability, partnerships
NHS Trusts GPs Foundation Trusts Private sector	PCTs – commissioning services from NHS Trusts, GPs, Foundation Trust and private companies: local partnership; GP contracts

If we start first with structure and look at the left hand part of this figure we can see at the base the service providers – the Trusts, which ran the hospitals, mental health, community and ambulance services; GPs with their primary care teams; and later the Foundation Trusts and private sector organisations.

Moving upwards it shows that the GPs were accountable for the performance of contracts agreed by PCTs; whilst both Trusts and PCTs were directly accountable to the SHAs. The SHAs, in turn, together with the Department of Health and some of the central bodies such as the MA were accountable to the Chief Executive and Permanent Secretary (CE/PS) who was in turn accountable to the Secretary of State (S of S) for delivery and policy development and to Parliament for expenditure. The S of S had some central bodies such as NICE account to him whilst others such as CHI were accountable to Parliament. This diagram ignores the complexity of relationships between S of S, Prime Minister, Chancellor, Cabinet, Parliament and the Head of State.

Over time some Trusts became Foundation Trusts and were no longer accountable to the SHAs but were regulated by Monitor.

On the processes side the figure shows that accountability flows upwards to Parliament which is able to hold the S of S to account on the floor of the House of Commons and in Committee, call the CE/PS to the Public Accounts Committee on expenditure and receive reports from the new regulators. The S of S is appointed by the Prime Minister and part of the Cabinet. The CE/PS is responsible to the S of S for implementation of policy and to work with him on policy development and budget setting. Together the S of S and the CE/PS chaired the Modernisation Board.

Timeline of key events

1948 – Foundation of NHS

1985 – Griffiths Report introducing general management into the NHS

1991 – First NHS Trusts established

1994 – Primary care led NHS

1997 – Election leads to Labour Government

Changes to PFI which make it viable

1998 – Quality framework agreed leading to establishment of NICE and CHI

Announcement of establishment of NHS Direct

2000 – PCTs established in three waves over succeeding years

NHS Plan Published

Chief Executive and Permanent Secretary appointed

Comprehensive Spending Review giving four year increased budgets from 2001

2001 – Modernisation Agency established

Shifting the Balance of power – giving main major role to PCTS

General Election

First Star Ratings introduced

Top Team established

2002 – First improved results published in Chief Executive's Report

Wanless report published

Delivering the NHS Plan published initiating system reforms

Use of private sector contractors permitted

2003 – Introduction of payment by results, increased patient choice, Independent Sector Treatment Centres

John Reid becomes Secretary of State

Introduction of new Consultant and GP Contracts

2004 – Monitor, regulator of Foundation Trusts, established and first Foundation Trusts authorised

Choosing Health white paper published

New target of 18 weeks from referral to treatment

Publication of NHS Improvement Plan

Introduction of Agenda for change

MRSA target agreed

First LIFT premises opened

Figures published showing private patients numbers reduced

2005 – A patient led NHS published:

Independence, Well being and Choice: Our Vision for the future of Social Care for Adults in England published

Election: Patricia Hewitt becomes Secretary of State

A Commissioning led NHS published initiating reorganisation

Major NHS targets achieved on time at end of year

2006 – *Our health, our care, our say: a new direction for community services* published
NHS overspends

2007 – NHS returns to financial balance

2008 – Ara Darzi's *"Next Steps Review"* published

2009 – Care Quality Commission established covering health and social care

2010 – "best practice tariffs" introduced for payment by results: 18 week waiting and MRSA targets achieved

Appendix 4

"Must do" targets in the NHS Plan pages 130–132

For the NHS

- reduce the maximum wait for an outpatient appointment to 3 months and the maximum wait for inpatient treatment to 6 months by the end of 2005
- patients will receive treatment at a time that suits them in accordance with their clinical need: two thirds of all outpatient appointments and inpatient elective admissions will be pre-booked by 2003/04 on the way to 100% pre-booking by 2005
- guaranteed access to a primary care professional within 24 hours and to a primary care doctor within 48 hours by 2004
- to secure year-on-year improvements in patient satisfaction including standards of cleanliness and food as measured by independently audited surveys
- reduce substantially the mortality rates from major killers by 2010; from heart disease by at least 40% in people under 75; from cancer by at least 20% in people under 75; and from suicide and undetermined injury by at least 20%. Key to the delivery of this target will be implementing the National Service Frameworks for Coronary Heart Disease, and Mental Health and the National Cancer Plan
- our objective is to narrow the health gap in childhood and throughout life between socio-economic groups and between the most deprived areas and the rest of the country. Specific national targets will be developed with stakeholders and experts early in 2001
- the cost of care commissioned from trusts which perform well against indicators of fair access, quality and responsiveness will become the benchmark for the NHS. Everyone will be expected to reach the level of the best over the next five years, with agreed milestones for 2003/04.

For the **NHS** in partnership with social services

- provide high quality pre-admission and rehabilitation care to older people to help them live as independently as possible by reducing preventable hospitalisation and ensuring year-on-year reductions in delays in moving people over 75 on from hospital. We expect at least 130,000 people to benefit and we will monitor progress in the Performance Assessment Framework

- increase the participation of problem drug users in drug treatment programmes by 55% by 2004, and 100% by 2008.

For Social Services

Improve the life chances for children in care by:

- improving the level of education, training and employment outcomes for care leavers aged 19, so that levels for this group are at least 75% of those achieved by all young people in the same area by March 2004

- increasing the percentage of children in care who achieve at least five grade A* to C GCSEs to 15% by 2004

- giving them the care and guidance needed to narrow the gap by 2004 between the proportion of children in care and their peers who are cautioned or convicted

- maximising the contribution adoption can make to providing permanent families for children; a specific target will be set in the light of the Prime Minister's review of adoption services.

Acknowledgements

I am particularly grateful to John Bacon, David Percy and Susana Edjang who have read almost all these chapters in draft and generously offered their comments and advice. They have improved the book.

I am also very grateful to a large number of people who have given me their reflections and, in many cases, let me quote them. They have included Sir George Alberti, John Appleby, Louis Appleby, Cristian Baeza, Vivian Bazalgette, Dame Chris Beasley, Helen Bevan, Maureen Bisognano, Harry Cayton, Yvonne Coghill, Peter Coates, Dame Sally Davies, Mike Deegan, Sir Andrew Dillon, Jennifer Dixon, Sir Liam Donaldson, Richard Douglas, Ruth English, David Fillingham, Andrew Foster, Phil Freeman, Richard Granger, Sir Muir Gray, Sian Jarvis, David Jenkins, Chris Liddle, Lord Andrew Mawson, Al Mulley, Sir John Oldham, Ariel Pablos-Mendez, Dean Royles, Paddy Salmon, and Keith Willett.

I should also like to put on record my gratitude and appreciation of a number of people who taught me so much about leadership and management both before I came to the NHS and in my early days as an NHS Manager. I have learned an enormous amount from Derek Adams, Michael Martindale, Peter Bagnall and Sir Brian Smith in particular.

As Chief Executive and Permanent Secretary I was wonderfully supported by many colleagues and by a succession of Principal Private Secretaries including Ruth Wetterstadt, Mark Davies, Dave McNeil, Shaun Gallagher and Ruth Cuthbert. Kate Barnard and Penny Jones provided coaching and wise counsel throughout the period and Judy Sweeting made sure I was always where I needed to be.

Above all I am grateful to Siân for reading all these chapters — her comments have been invaluable — and to her, Madeleine and Alastair for their love and forbearance.

Nigel Crisp
July 2011

Index